MEDICINE MOMS™

MEDICINE MOMS™

*Reclaiming Our Children's
Health Through Homeopathy
and Common Sense*

Arlene Uhl

Foreword by Luc De Schepper, M.D.

TWIN STREAMS
KENSINGTON PUBLISHING CORP.
http://www.kensingtonbooks.com

The names and identifying details of the parents and children in this book have been altered to protect privacy.

This book is in no way meant as a substitute for professional medical consultation.

KENSINGTON BOOKS are published by

Kensington Publishing Corp.
850 Third Avenue
New York, NY 10022

All Kensington titles, imprints and distributed lines are available at special quantity discounts for bulk purchases for sales promotion, premiums, fund raising, educational or institutional use.

Special book excerpts or customized printings can also be created to fit specific needs. For details, write or phone the office of the Kensington Special Sales Manager: Kensington Publishing Corp., 850 Third Avenue, New York, NY, 10022. Attn. Special Sales Department. Phone: 1-800-221-2647.

Kensington and the K logo Reg. U.S. Pat. & TM Off.
Twin Streams and TS are trademarks of Kensington Publishing Corp.

ISBN 1-57566-645-6

First Printing: March, 2001
10 9 8 7 6 5 4 3 2 1

Printed in the United States of America

For
Lauren Bartel

CONTENTS

FOREWORD

Behind almost every conversion to modalities like acupuncture and homeopathy lies an anecdote—here's mine. When I graduated from medical school, I felt like a combination of Dr. Schweitzer and Superman: my suitcase loaded full of injections of which I really knew little, my heart full of good intentions, my enthusiasm at a zenith point. Before I saw my first patient, I instructed my wife that in the event such a poor soul showed up, she should tell him that I was very busy and let him wait a little. It never looks good to seem like you have just been sitting around waiting for a patient! When later that same day the doorbell rang, hopes were high: the first catch of the day! My wife rushed down the stairs while I tried to hide. Having been well instructed, she said to the man at the door, "My husband will be right with you, he is talking on the phone with a patient." The man looked puzzled and then replied slowly, "That's very strange. I'm from the phone company and came to install the phone." What an embarrassment! However, my painful journey was not finished yet. My first real patient was a young girl, fifteen years old, suffering from chronic headaches. The headache was frequently triggered by a change of weather—which was unfortunate, as the weather changed four times a day in Belgium. She had been given all the existing headache medications from previous doctors but she thought as I was this new young gun, I must have some new weapons in my arsenal. Of course I had none. After the telephone and headache debacle, I took an aspirin for my own headache, and decided there and then that there must be life beyond allopathy, as we call Western medicine. That was twenty-eight years ago, and I can honestly say I have never stopped studying since. I discarded all my original medical books and replaced them with acupuncture and homeopathy books. To this day I have not regretted this change. On the contrary, I have earned far more gratitude and appreciation and derived far more satisfaction than I ever could have dreamt of securing by doling out routine prescriptions of allopathic medicine.

Many among us might think that Western medicine has reached the pinnacle of scientific achievement, from which it will proceed from triumph to triumph. But medicine suffers from several defects which, unless remedied, may halt its further progress. There is first of all a lack of individualization. Western medical books are like catalogues describing diseases. We doctors try very hard to fit each patient into one such category, so that the omnipresent protocol will take care of the illness. On top of that, in allopathy there are no laws and principles by which to gauge if the patient is really doing better or worse. I have seen so many patients who felt really miserable and had normal lab results; while there are doctors who tell their patients who are feeling fine that they really ought to feel bad because their lab results have gone up two points. A homeopathic physician never tries to put the name of a disease on a patient. We don't have diseases, we have *patients with* diseases! We have patients with arthritis, diabetes, hypertension . . . not arthritis, diabetes, and hypertension coming for a visit. Homeopathy is a scientific method based on thousands of years of observation of Nature. A physician will never be led astray if he sticks to these principles. *Our first duty is to the truth, which, when loyally served, best enables us to do the greatest good to the sick.*

Second of all, have the wonders of Western medicine been uniformly wonderful? New drugs, new vaccinations, new genetic discoveries, new techniques to probe deeper and deeper in the human body . . . these accomplishments are indeed impressive.

Yet there is disturbing news on the horizon. Since World War II infectious diseases have been considered on the verge of eradication; in fact, Secretary of State George Marshall made a speech to that effect in 1948. Yet today, they are the number one cause of death in the world, and old-fashioned diseases like whooping cough, TB, and cholera are coming back in record numbers. Microbes are becoming more and more resistant, due in part to the flagrant overuse of antibiotics by medical doctors and factory farms. These antibiotics, which we thought would eradicate infectious diseases in our lifetime, are becoming increasingly powerless against the new strains of resistant bacteria. Diarrhea, which we think of as a relatively harmless infectious disease, kills millions of children worldwide every year, making it the second leading cause of death after cardiovascular disease. Tuberculosis, malaria, diarrhea, and sexually transmitted diseases are the real silent epidemics. Our attention may be diverted by the horror stories about AIDS and the Ebola virus, but these silent epidemics affect far more people. Conventional medicine is touted as the leader in the management of infectious diseases. Yet homeopathy has always been more successful against the great epidemic diseases: cholera, typhoid fever, diphtheria, scarlet fever. In the great flu epidemic in the early twentieth century, the statistics in London hospitals showed the mortality rate at allopathic hospitals was 55 percent, but less than 5 percent at homeopathic hospitals.

Medical practices outside of "official" medicine have always been an important part of the public's health care. In fact, until the early decades of this century, allopathic medicine coexisted with homeopathic and herbal medicine in this country, as it still does in nearly every other country in the world. In fact, I know of no other country in which one form of medicine has such a monopoly of legal protection and insurance reimbursement as allopathic medicine does in this country. Alternative healers, through the centuries, have offered a multiplicity of ways to address the confusion and suffering that accompany disease. The notion of alternative medicine as quackery (a term originally applied to *allopathic* physicians for using toxic doses of mercury to "cure" syphilis) has been reinforced by a once commonly heard definition of it as any treatment not taught in an accredited medical school. This definition is no longer valid, as most medical schools have added nontraditional courses in response to growing public interest in alternative therapies. With this change in attitude came a change in name to *complementary* or *integrative* medicine, indicating that allopathy and alternative methods can be used together to support each other.

While we are seeing tremendous interest in complementary medicine among the public—and a slow but increasing interest among medical doctors—we still have a long way to go. One mistake I see among allopathic practitioners is to lump all the different forms of nonallopathic healing into one basket. But certain forms—notably acupuncture, homeopathy, and chiropractic—require years of study of health sciences comparable to the years of training in conventional medicine, and they should not be lumped together with psychic healers, pendulum dowsers, and tarot card readers. This does a disservice to forms of healing that are based on scientific laws and principles and that merit the serious inquiry of the open-minded allopath.

In my lectures about homeopathy at medical schools and hospitals, certain issues keep coming up, especially the argument that homeopathy, like herbal and other "eclectic" medicines, is an old-fashioned form of healing, practiced by people with little to no training, regulation of practice, or standards for quality of care. Let's look at the facts. It is true that in allopathic medicine we certainly would not accept any drug or procedure from more than fifty years ago (and most drugs are out of date within a few years), but to me it is a strength of homeopathy that we use the same remedies discovered when homeopathy was founded nearly two hundred years ago. When a new drug comes out, often side effects and serious problems are discovered only when millions of people start using it. It gives me confidence in homeopathy to know that the remedies have already been used by millions of people worldwide for many decades, and their effects are well known. Our knowledge in homeopathy keeps building and building on strong solid scientific principles; we do not have to keep discarding what we know as allopathic medicine does.

Furthermore, in the nineteenth century, when homeopathy enjoyed widespread support especially among the educated classes, homeopathic physicians received the same training as their allopathic colleagues *plus* an additional two years of homeopathy. It was well known that the most brilliant medical students would go on to become homeopaths. Unfortunately the pressure from allopathic medical societies in the early years of the twentieth century, plus the lure of the "magic bullet" of the new antibiotic drugs, soon led to a decline in homeopathy to the point that twenty years ago very few medical doctors were practicing it. The old guard had almost all died off and very few new doctors were joining. With the rise of interest in alternative medicine a quarter-century ago, the gap was filled at first with lay homeopaths. Now we have a tremendous interest in homeopathy among MDs, osteopaths, naturopaths, veterinarians, nurse practitioners, chiropractors, and acupuncturists. I can see this in my own school, where dozens of health care professionals are learning to incorporate homeopathy into their practices.

What about the question of research? So often we see in the popular press—and even in medical journals, whose authors should know better—that homeopathy is "unproven" and "there is no scientific evidence to support it." The fact is that homeopathy does have good scientific evidence to back it up. And the meta-analyses (overviews of all the studies on homeopathy) have shown that the better designed the study, the more likely it was to demonstrate the effectiveness of homeopathy. Within the past few years some good research on homeopathy has been done in this country and published in mainstream medical journals. With the government finally funding research, we can look forward to more of it in the years to come.

I have no problem with my allopathic colleagues scrutinizing the potential risks and benefits of alternative medicine. Let's examine some of them and see if homeopathy can pass muster.

Quality of care is often the first argument brought up by my colleagues. Homeopathy definitely has the potential to provide the same (or better) quality of care as allopathic medicine. In the past, as we mentioned, the most brilliant physicians were the homeopaths, and homeopathic licensure had the same components as allopathic licensure (in terms of the content and length of training, testing and certification, a defined scope of practice, review and audit, and codified disciplinary action). The fact that homeopathy does not currently have this licensure system is due to the political and economic forces at work in this country, not a reflection on homeopathy itself. Licensure efforts for homeopathy are underway in a number of states, at the same time that an increasing number of already-licensed professionals are incorporating homeopathy into their practices. In other words, this objection is only a temporary one until the United States can catch up with Europe, the former Soviet States, and India in providing professional training and licensure for homeopaths.

Quality of products is another potential argument against alternative modalities. Random tests of vitamins, supplements, and herbs often show that the contents do not measure up to what is on the label. Nor do the labels contain adequate warnings about the potentially toxic effects of large overdoses of some of those supplements. But homeopathic remedies are completely safe, nontoxic, and very inexpensive, and unlike prescription drugs, homeopathic remedies are prescribed *one* at a time, thereby avoiding possible dangerous interactions. We must not forget that 100,000 deaths a year in this country are caused by conventional drugs.

Quality of science is probably one of the main allopathic arguments. Allopathic medicine claims to be based on the double-blind method, and discredits any form of alternative medicine that cannot fully support every remedy or procedure with double-blind research studies. Yet allopathic medicine itself violates this principle every day; surgeries, for example, are difficult to test by this method. And according to allopathic research, 67 percent of all drugs are prescribed on the basis of a "secondary use," that is, a side effect—in other words, not according to the original double-blind protocol.

Without any doubt, homeopathy could be advanced by organized professional standards and greater availability of instruction to interested health care professionals. That the public has embraced alternative medicine has been proven by the excellent 1998 study by David Eisenberg of Harvard Medical School, which indicated that 70 percent of the population had consulted an alternative practitioner. Because of its great results in the past and present, homeopathy will undoubtedly catch the attention of patients ready to embrace a scientific approach that has proven its validity in the last two hundred years. I hope that allopathic physicians will show a serious interest in this marvelous approach before they reject it. Humankind will be the better for it!

Why do I like *Medicine Moms*?

Because it is the journey of an intelligent mom who, like many others, was disenchanted with the shot-gun approach of allopathy. Her book approaches the subject of homeopathy with an objective, analytical mind, based on the author's in-depth study and research, validating the initial positive findings of the homeopathic approach to her child with other's people experiences, and with more scientific data as well.

I like this book because it demonstrates beautifully the difference between the homeopathic physician's approach and the allopath: the homeopath looking at a patient *with* a disease, the allopath trying to classify all patients under a singular disease name so he can resort to the protocol, easy to administer and comforting. But comforting to whom? Mainly to the allopathic physician.

I like this book because it guides the reader to find an appropriate homeopathic physician by asking the right questions. As in any profession, there is a great variety in quality. This book will make a choice easier. Your family deserves the best!

I like this book because it guides the reader to try well-proven remedies in every day *acute* situations. The successful use of some of these acute remedies will then bring the reader to the professional homeopath to find out if there is "something that can be done for this chronic condition" (which *always* should be addressed by a homeopathic physician!).

And I like it because it tells the reader how to cross over that bridge to "break" the news to your family, friends, and allopathic physician, that you have now entered a different modality with its own logical way of thinking.

Best of all, this book without any doubt will arouse the curiosity of its many readers to try homeopathy and study its effects. Therefore *Medicine Moms* has a place in every family's library!

Dr. Luc De Schepper
San Diego

INTRODUCTION

Greetings from a Medicine Mom

A man could not be born alive and healthy were there not already a physician in him.

—Paracelsus, sixteenth-century physician

I am not a medical doctor, and I don't even play one on television.

I am not a New Age "flake." I do not worship comets, hug trees, or make my own granola. I have never been abducted by aliens.

The women you'll hear about in this book—the growing ranks of Medicine Moms—are pretty much like me. They are not militants or radicals, or anarchists or survivalists. Heck, they don't have time to be any kind of "—ists." They pilot station wagons and minivans, plan birthday parties, read bedtime stories, treat boo-boos with TLC (and the movie tie-in Band-Aid of the week), help with the homework, do too much laundry, and do it all because they really care about their families. They are your basic card-carrying millennial moms. And the only flakes in their houses are made from corn (okay, and occasionally bran).

As for our kids, well, you know them too. They are cartoon-ogling, Gameboy-toting, soccer-playing, karate-kicking, cookie-craving, Brussels sprout-loathing, twenty-first-century munchkins. They love dinosaurs, Barbies, assorted odd Japanese monsters, cute but overpriced stuffed animals, and—oh, yes—Elmo and friends. They hate it when they feel sick. (What fun is that?) And we—their moms—find it's no picnic for us either.

Whatever differences our families may have, one powerful idea connects us. We want our kids (and—not incidentally—ourselves) to be healthy and happy.

That's the simple reason why we, a bunch of mainstream, Main

Street mothers (and, yes, many dads as well) have become disenchanted with certain aspects of conventional medicine. That's why we have gradually begun taking increased responsibility for the health of our loved ones and spreading the word among our neighbors, relations, and friends. That's why we have become part of a burgeoning grass roots American movement exploring homeopathy, a system of medicine that is gentle, efficient, and—hallelujah! —often effective where more invasive methods (e.g., antibiotics, steroid inhalants, and those "tubes in the ears") have repeatedly failed us.

As this book will explain in detail, homeopathy is not new, nor is it considered literally "alternative" in many places. It is widely integrated into mainstream health care in much of the rest of the world, including Western Europe. It is based on sound empirical science with more and more studies appearing to support its validity every year. And it is currently enjoying a well-deserved second look by many former skeptics.

In the 1990s, the proportion of the U.S. population that used homeopathy quintupled, bringing it to several million.[1] And in roughly the same period of time, worldwide sales of homeopathic products increased more than tenfold, to more than a billion dollars annually.[2] Undoubtedly we Medicine Moms are helping these statistics swell.

Why are we playing such a large role in resurrecting a system that dates back two hundred years and which predates our modern medical "miracles"? The answer is simple: because it works.

This book is the story of what we have learned, what all parents can learn, and what more are learning every day. Best of all, it is a happy story—one not just of healing, but of life enhancement and personal empowerment.

If your interest is piqued, please read on. Perhaps one day soon, aspects of it will be part of your story as well.

CHAPTER
1

Mommy, Where Did My Cough Go?

The Lord hath created medicines out of the earth; and he that is wise will not abhor them.

—Ecclesiasticus, *Apocryphe*

God could not be everywhere and therefore he made mothers.

—Jewish proverb

I remember bringing my son home from the hospital soon after he was born. He looked so tiny and vulnerable, and I felt so protective. I could hardly wait for my first pediatrician's appointment so I could assure myself that I was doing a good job and everything was "normal."

In a few days, the big moment came. My husband and I bundled up our bundle and took him into the doctor's office, where he was briskly and professionally weighed, measured, prodded, poked, and returned to us with instructions:

"Don't take him anywhere for two months," said the doctor. "He might catch something."

This advice took us aback somewhat. For one thing, it put a crimp in our plans to stop at the A&P on the way home. And what about him getting a little fresh air now and again? After all, spring was in bloom and the breeze was gentle and warm. Nevertheless, I went home and dutifully called a friend of mine to cancel plans to take our babies for an outing in a local park the following week.

My friend thought this was the funniest thing she'd ever heard. She was a mother of three herself, and would have found taking my pediatrician's advice impossible unless she was prepared to quarantine her four-year-old and six-year-old for the next few months while she and her baby stayed at home. Moreover, she thought it was, well, a bit extreme.

She would not presume to tell me what to do, of course, but our conversation did get me to thinking. Somehow the human race has prospered for millennia without barricading babies off from other humans. What would a prehistoric cave mom have replied to my doctor's eight-week dictum: "Ugh"?

But then again, Cave Mom did not grow up in a society where questioning "doctor's orders" was considered sacrilege. All she had to rely on were other cave moms, her own experience, and her wits. Whereas I had all the benefits of modern medical knowledge.

I pondered some more. The days grew warmer. Ultimately, I stopped pondering and took my baby to the park—and he survived!

Although at the time I did not consciously realize it, a sea change had begun in my outlook. Perhaps, just perhaps, the word of a pediatrician was not always to be confused with the Word of a deity. And perhaps, as a mother, I could begin—ever so gradually—to trust my own instincts.

I later would refer to this as Phase One of my own private epiphany.

Phase Two was equally as subtle.

Thankfully, I was blessed with a healthy baby. Indeed, for the first year of his life, the only problem that cropped up was the routine one of teething pains. But none of the usual over-the-counter medications that were recommended seemed to help. My poor boy would endure paroxysms of wailing misery night after night. I despaired of finding anything that would ease his frustration, not to mention my own.

Then one evening, a colleague called to chat, and heard—how could she not?—my baby in the background sending up his customary siren. "Teething?" she guessed, for she herself had a son a few months older than mine. "Don't tell me you haven't tried *chamomilla* tablets."

"Huh?" said I.

Chamomilla tablets, she explained, were made from the chamomile plant. They worked like a charm on teething woes, she asserted, and, furthermore, they were safe and gentle because they were homeopathic.

I had no idea what "homeopathic" meant. But I'd had chamomile tea, which was sort of soothing, and I figured I'd just give this stuff a try. As per my colleague's instructions I went to my local health food store and got a bottle of these tablets in "melt-away" form, so they could dissolve easily on a baby's tongue.

Home I went to administer them and—hello?—did someone say "miracle"? I kid you not, within minutes after popping one of these innocuous little tabs on my son's tongue, his drooling and bright red facial flush subsided, his screeching halted, and his face broke out in a big (toothy) grin.

I thought at first it was a coincidence, but it just kept on happening. From then on, when he'd get worked up, it was *chamomilla* time, and that was the end of that.

Over the next few days, these results were validated by an interested third party—my husband—whose newfound ability to get a good night's sleep made him an early convert to homeopathy's seeming magic. But then, of course, I met my first skeptic.

At that time I was working outside my home two days a week, seeing my psychotherapy patients. I had a wonderful babysitter on those days, and of course I explained to her what she should now do if the "teething meanies" showed up. Although she looked at me like I was a few cards shy of a deck, she agreed to give it a try. By the time I called to check in later that afternoon, she was wonderstruck. "My goodness," she said, "I'll never go to work without *this* in my bag again." In the background, my son giggled contentedly.

Soon enough, of course, the teething crisis passed, and the little white tablets made their way to the back of the medicine cabinet, behind the oft-forgotten vitamins and last summer's sunscreen. I never did find out what "homeopathic" meant, and life went on.

Again, I consider myself extremely lucky. My son was rarely ill. For this I was thankful, not only for the obvious reason that all of us wish our children the best of health, but also because I was beginning to notice, all around me, what seemed to be a strange phenomenon. So many of my friends and neighbors with small children were having an awful time of it health-wise.

The pattern seemed to be that a child would come down with a cold, be taken to the pediatrician, diagnosed with an ear infection, and be put on antibiotics. Then, a few weeks later, the entire scenario would repeat itself. And so it would continue to go, until it seemed, as many of them commented, that both the infections and the antibiotics had become a way of life.

It seemed odd to them, and to me. But I didn't pay too much attention until at age two and a half, my child—now in a part-time nursery school program—began to succumb.

First it was a cold, then it was a persistent cough, then it was a fever high enough so that I took him in to the doctor who proclaimed he had an ear infection. Then it was amoxicillin, the pink bacteria-slaying goo with which nearly every contemporary mom is now all too familiar. Then it was amoxicillin again, because it didn't work the first time. Then it was a broad-spectrum antibiotic (i.e., a more vigilant bacteria slayer). Then—because that didn't work either, it was time for Phase Three of my epiphany to begin.

I began to do a little research, read a few things, browse around the Web. It seems some highly credible and mainstream sources were maintaining that antibiotics were overused and that for some conditions, e.g., ear infections, they were also largely ineffective.

With my heart literally pounding in my ears from nerves, I dared to question my child's doctor.

"Um, you know," I ventured timidly, "I've been reading where, er, maybe these back-to-back courses of antibiotics can do more harm than good. You know, compromise the immune system. Do you think we could just give him two weeks and see if the body clears this up by itself? You know, I think it was in the *Journal of the American Medical Association* . . ."

But I noticed the doctor wasn't listening any longer. Instead, he was looking at me like I had sprouted another head, and it was neon green. "That's ridiculous," he practically shouted. "Why, I would try four or five different kinds of antibiotics before trying something like *that.*"

Oh. Okay. "Well, what about preventive measures?" I meekly posed. If one of those four or five other drugs did clear this up, was there anything I could do to prevent it from coming back?

My neon head apparently grew brighter, because it was really drawing an incredulous stare. "Preventive!" he scoffed. He scribbled another prescription and with that I was, evidently, dismissed. I left with my poor, miserable, earlobe-tugging tot in tow.

Now, I have to take a moment here and say that I have, before and since this incident, encountered and been told of many estimable, reasonable, open-minded, and compassionate physicians. Moreover this book is not a diatribe against the medical profession, but an invitation for all of us—layperson and medical professional, parent and doctor—to join together in the name of health. But this particular incident was highly unsettling and unsatisfying to say the least.

I once read a quote by the diarist Alice James, sister of novelist Henry and philosopher William James, in which she said: "I suppose one has a greater sense of intellectual degradation after an interview with a doctor than from any human experience."[1] At the moment I left our pediatrician's office that day, I knew exactly what Alice meant.

So there I was clutching a prescription I really didn't want to fill. But could I possibly *not* fill it without feeling as though I was taking a risk with the thing most precious to me—my own child's well-being?

I forestalled my decision while foraging in my local supermarket. And right then, fate intervened, as it is sometimes wont to do, pointing me in a new direction. For there, by the frozen chicken nuggets, I encountered an old friend I hadn't seen in a while. I told her what was new with me and she, in turn, told me a story. Before I continue with my own, let me tell you hers.

Ginny's Story

Ginny is the mother of two lovely little girls. I had known that her eldest, Leah, then three years old, had quite a bout with recurrent ear infections. But because I hadn't seen Ginny in a while, I had not known that her two-year-old, Stacey, had developed the same problem, as well as severe allergies.

Stacey had been having an extraordinarily difficult time the previous spring, Ginny said, because she could barely breathe through her nose at night. Since she sucked her thumb for comfort, breathing properly through her mouth was also difficult. This made for many long and sleepless vigils. None of the usual medications, either over-the-counter or prescription, did much to alleviate the problem, but clearly something had to be done. Ginny said it "broke her heart" to think of giving a two-year-old allergy shots, so she asked her pediatrician if there wasn't any other possible alternative.

Her doctor, whom she liked and trusted, also seemed to feel exasperated. He told Ginny that he had heard, via a pharmacist in the area who was knowledgeable about homeopathic medicines and kept his establishment well stocked with them, that a homeopathic physician had just begun a practice in a nearby town. Ginny promptly made an appointment.

"He gave Stacey a remedy," Ginny said. "From the first night she was on it, Stacey could breathe through her nose!"

As for those ear infections, the next time both girls came down with them, Ginny decided to try calling the homeopath again. "I had bought a homeopathic home care kit, on a whim. And the doctor told me what I needed was in it. I gave them some *belladonna,* and held my breath. I was scared, you see. It felt weird to be doing this, instead of dosing the kids with Tylenol®. But their fevers came down. I kept up the homeopathic treatment and, the way the doctor explained it to me, it just helped them heal themselves."

By the time I ran into Ginny that day, it was six months since she'd met this homeopathic doctor. In the interim she, her husband,

and her mother had all visited him for various chronic complaints. The family had never been healthier, she vowed. It was quite an amazing thing.

My "Aha!" Experience

Ginny, it's important to say, didn't pressure me in any way. It was clear she was an enthusiastic "satisfied customer" of homeopathy, but she did not try to convert me or recruit me into something for which I wasn't ready. However, I truly was intrigued. At the very least, I figured finding out more couldn't hurt. Besides, I seemed to recall positively that word "homeopathic." Wasn't that what those little miracle teething tablets had been called?

So I called the homeopath, and arranged for us to be seen as soon as possible, taking the first cancellation that came along. Before he saw us, though, he required that I fill out a lengthy questionnaire all about my son's health, habits, disposition, and so on. I already had a good feeling about this, because it seemed like this homeopath really wanted to understand my kid, and not just his germs.

At that first appointment, the doctor explained, in simple terms, how homeopathic medicines were made from infinitesimal doses of natural substances which served to stimulate or enhance the body's own natural ability to restore and maintain good health. I was to find out a great deal more about the details as time went on, but right then I just wanted my son to get over his ear infections.

The doctor prescribed one remedy, *thuja* (a plant from the Coniferae family), which was meant to counteract any adverse effects of antibiotics, and another, *belladonna,* to treat the acute aspects of the ear condition itself. *Belladonna,* as it turns out, is a plant whose name means *beautiful woman,* so called because in times past women would wash their face with it to give them a healthy blush. Later, as I came to understand more about homeopathy and learn the Law of Similars which guides it, it would become clear why one would prescribe this for a condition that involved fever and face flushing. But at that moment, I was simply hoping it would do the job.

And so it did. My son's condition cleared up nicely. And the next time—perhaps a month later—when he woke up from a nap all flushed and crying "Ear hurt," I was ready. I checked with the homeopath right away, administered *belladonna,* and watched it work its wonders again. Within less than an hour, my son's normal temperature and temperament were restored.

"Aha!" I thought. "I think I'm on to something here."

What's more, the best was yet to come. After working with my practitioner for a few months, he gave my son a remedy that he termed his "constitutional." (In my child's case, it was *sulphur,* but constitutionals vary depending on the overall physical and emotional picture of each unique individual.) A constitutional, my doctor explained, is in effect the final layer of the onion. Given after acute problems are resolved, it is meant to strengthen the overall system and prevent recurrence of illness. As was predicted, after my son received his homeopathic dose of the mineral *sulphur,* episodes of colds, ear infections, and so on were far less frequent and far less severe. In fact, that winter, while his classmates succumbed to the usual array of cold weather illnesses in droves, my boy had barely a sniffle.

Was I happy? You bet. But you know, when you're a parent, it's always something.

Along with my happiness came a certain measure of self-doubt. Sure this all seemed well and good but . . . was I sure I was doing the best thing for my child? What, exactly, was I putting in his system? How was it made? Had homeopathy been thoroughly researched and tested?

The truth is, I wasn't sure. Now, I don't like being unsure. So I undertook the cure for uncertainty: I got a lot of information.

Back to books I went, and off to some seminars my homeopathic physician was giving for parents and health professionals both. Of course, too, back to the Internet, where I found a wealth of

enlightening and comforting information not only from such helpful organizations as the National Center for Homeopathy but also
from the most mainstream of medical publications. Several of the
latter were beginning to report on the effectiveness of homeopathy
when tested by the gold standard of scientific research—the
double-blind controlled placebo-study (the kind where neither researchers nor subjects know who is receiving a medication versus
who is receiving a placebo).

Knowing these things helped give me peace of mind, and added
courage to my convictions. Although I was hardly becoming a cru-
sader, I no longer felt sheepish about answering questions posed to
me by friends and neighbors who had gotten wind of the fact my
family was doing something a bit out of the ordinary.

"What's that stuff you use?" people would ask tentatively, when
they noticed my son circumventing the winter flu and then sailing
relatively unscathed through a brutal spring and summer hayfever
season.

"Who's that homeopath? Is he a *real* doctor?"

"How does this work again?"

And I would tell them some of what I knew, while careful never
to be a "pusher." (Because who doesn't hate that?)

Sure, some of those I discussed homeopathy with looked at me
like I had a bone in my nose. But as the old saying goes, nothing
succeeds like success—and firsthand evidence. Slowly but surely,
as more mothers grew frustrated with the same old unsatisfactory
solutions to their children's health complaints, there began to be a
grass roots movement in my circle of acquaintance.

One by one, like dominoes, many of the women I knew became interested in exploring options for managing their family's
health. In an increasing number of households, tiny white homeopathic pellets replaced antibacterial pink goo. And at the local
playgrounds, the swapping of information on this compelling subject replaced (or at least supplemented) the usual topics of T-ball
sign-up and phonics versus whole word reading.

Now I don't mean to suggest we just went off half-cocked and started treating our children's illnesses without professional consultation. We readily availed ourselves of *all* resources. Still, this phenomenon made me think of what it must have been like generations ago, when women relied on each other's common sense and practical experience in order to preserve the good health of their loved ones. Each one in turn freely tapped into that body of wisdom, becoming a wellspring for those who followed her.

Such medicine women may belong to history, but in my neck of the woods, the Medicine Mom had arrived.

Katie's Story

Now remember the babysitter I mentioned—the one who was so pleasantly startled by the effect of *chamomilla* on my son's teething pains? By now she had her own baby daughter, Maria.

Shortly after Maria was born, Katie had gone to purchase a bottle of *chamomilla* tablets to have on hand. She ended up buying a set of about a dozen homeopathic remedies, all of which were meant to be useful in treating minor childhood ailments. She put those other remedies on the kitchen shelf, where they sat untouched for some time, and pretty much forgot about them.

When Maria first came down with an ear infection, Katie did not think twice about giving her daughter the prescribed antibiotics. And they seemed to work just fine.

But when another ear infection came along shortly thereafter, the same antibiotic didn't work at all. So another was prescribed. Another infection, another antibiotic, and so on. The last medication in the series was, as Katie says, "a thick, smelly concoction that Maria hated to take." Perhaps, Katie says, it would have been worth the discomfort if it worked, but alas it did not. After taking an entire course of it, Maria now was diagnosed with a double ear infection.

"By this time," Katie recalled, "I can honestly say my doctor herself was uncomfortable prescribing more antibiotics. I really got the impression she was trying to say, 'Look, I don't like doing this, but it's my job.'"

By this point, though, Katie couldn't bring herself to fill the prescription. She "pocketed" it, and decided to wait to see if the infection cleared up on its own. Then she remembered the plastic bottles on her kitchen shelf. She read the booklet that had come along with them and decided to try the ear infection remedies it mentioned. Because she wasn't exactly sure which of two was the better choice, she alternated both. The infection cleared up, as her own doctor confirmed.

"I told my doctor what I had done, and she didn't say anything," says Katie. "Her reaction was not to react. But she didn't say not to do it, or issue any warnings. I could just tell she didn't want to hear the ins and outs, so long as the end result was a good one."

Katie always put her faith in her pediatrician, and still does. But now she also uses homeopathy—about which she has learned much more, including how to pick the best remedy that matches her daughter's exact symptoms. And she hopes her daughter's pediatrician will want to know more about it one day.

Mommy, Where Did My Cough Go?

While all of this was going on, a neighbor of mine from down the road was having a terrible dilemma that involved her then four-year-old son, Pete. Pete suffered from allergies and related respiratory problems. He had been given a diagnosis of RAD, reactive airway disorder.

He'd had lots and lots of antibiotics over the years, but nothing helped what his mother called Pete's "juicy, smoker's cough." During one nasty allergy season, Pete was so congested he ended up at the hospital emergency room. At that point his mother was instructed in how to use a nebulizer and inhalant medications to help him breathe. She was told to use what came to be known as "Pete's machine" every four hours when he was symptomatic, especially during the height of allergy season.

Unfortunately the medication Pete was inhaling had him, as his mother says, "bouncing off the walls." After using his nebulizer and inhaling his medication, Pete routinely became restless and cranky, totally worked up. "Plus," as his mother says, "he still had the cough." Although "Pete's machine" did temporarily open up his airways, Corrine says, his mucous wasn't dissolving or coming up.

"Finally," says Corrine, "things got to the point where enough was enough. I was having a meltdown, and my son was out of control—and sounding like he'd just had a pack of cigarettes to boot. My husband had to agree that we needed to try something else."

But what else? Corrine, of course, had an inkling. Although—I swear—I never pushed the issue, I had mentioned to her how homeopathy had been helpful to my family. And one day when Corrine herself was suffering a very runny nose from allergies, she half jokingly had asked me if I had a remedy for her.

I gave her something called *Allium cepa,* which is simply a minute, homeopathic (i.e., highly diluted) dose of red onion.

She wondered how red onion, which typically *induces* tearing and drippy noses, could make her nose stop running. I explained that homeopathy treats *like with like.* (That indeed is how the word *homeopathy,* which means "similar suffering" is derived.)

Where traditional Western medicine (a.k.a allopathy) treats a symptom by suppressing it and sometimes inducing an opposite condition (e.g. those dry-you-out antihistamines to counter wet noses), homeopathy would use a substance likely to induce a similar symptom to the one being experienced. It introduces that substance into the body's system in an infinitesimal amount, which activates the body's own healing abilities.

My neighbor looked dubious. And to be fair, who wouldn't? It all sounds a bit odd at first, I'll admit. Nevertheless she took the remedy. One hour later she knocked on my door. Her nose had stopped running, and she had administered some *Allium cepa* tablets to her six-month-old as well. His nose was also now dry. "I want your homeopath's number," she said. "If this works, I want to see what else does."

So she made an appointment, but soon felt conflicted about keeping it. Was she being foolish? Then fate intervened for Corrine as well. She met another woman who told her of her own child's medical condition, which was nearly identical to Pete's, and his happy homeopathic outcome. Who was this other woman? She was herself a pediatric nurse! Needless to say, Corrine brought her son to his appointment after all.

Within weeks, Pete was far less dependent on his inhalants, and thriving. Homeopathy had a new fan, and a new source of information for other mothers. Now Corrine doesn't get up on a soapbox and shout about her newfound beliefs. But when the topic of health and well-being arises, she often tells the story of how Pete looked at her one day after his allergies had been brought under control and asked, "Mommy, where did my cough go?"

The Making of Medicine Moms

Where did Pete's cough go? Well, for one thing it went down in history in the annals of our neighborhood Medicine Moms as yet another example of how much can change when parents start empowering themselves and searching for viable options.

Our neighborhood saga is, of course, but one example. I share it with you in detail because it's the one I know best, but in researching this book, in attending gatherings of professionals and laypersons interested in homeopathy, in chatting on the Internet, and in just networking with friends and acquaintances—and their friends and acquaintances—across the country, I have encountered a myriad of people with stories so similar they sound like an old familiar refrain.

The fact is Medicine Moms are cropping up all over the place, without planning to or seeking to. What do we all have in common? Two things. First, we experienced a disillusionment with typical pediatric kid care.

We never expected to question our doctors, or challenge the status quo. Frankly, in the culture in which we grew up, we may have questioned other institutions, but certainly not the medical establishment. Even the most opinionated or iconoclastic among us wouldn't dream of arguing with science. We were conditioned to hold that sacrosanct. Besides, science was objective, wasn't it? So what was there to argue with?

But then we became parents. And once our children got involved in the medical system, sometimes things didn't seem so clear cut anymore.

We gave the conventional medical approach and those who practiced it every benefit of the doubt—until the doubt became completely overwhelming. We began to ask ourselves: What if our cars broke down every few weeks and we kept taking them back to the same mechanics, even though the mechanics never seemed to identify, let alone solve, the problem? And what if, in fact, those cars seemed to run a little worse, break down a bit sooner, after each visit to the auto shop? Would it make any sense to continue to turn to the same mechanics over and over again?

Reluctantly—and I say reluctantly because, after all, we wanted to believe in our mechanics, and it was still the path of least resistance to do so—we had to admit it would not.

But though disenchantment fueled our departure from the fold, it is only half the story. The second half brought new enchantment in the form of those "Aha!" experiences.

People familiar with homeopathy often half-jokingly use the phrase "conversion remedies." By this they are referring to the fact that most people who become regular users of homeopathy had at one point early on an experience of taking or administering a remedy that worked so quickly and precisely it knocked their proverbial socks off. It might be *belladonna* clearing up a string of recalcitrant ear infections; it might be *Allium cepa* turning off a perennial nose faucet; it might be *arnica,* another plant remedy whose astonishing effectiveness in easing the soreness of bruises, blunt traumas, and overexertion of muscles makes it a frequent "conversion remedy" for the sports enthusiast (or the mother of a sports enthusiast). Of course, it could be any remedy at all, but the point is those who are swayed by homeopathy generally tend to have an epiphany of this sort. It makes them think: Hey, if this is so powerful, what else is possible?

Interestingly enough, the disenchantment/enchantment cycle is often echoed by doctors who themselves become practitioners and advocates of homeopathy. Jennifer Jacobs, M.D., M.P.H., is a family physician in Edmonds, Washington, specializing in homeopathy. She is a past member of the advisory council of the National Institute of Health's Office of Alternative Medicine and the author of the first double-blind study on homeopathic medicines published in an American medical journal. Dr. Jacobs told me she became disillusioned during her residency when she saw that the side effects of many commonly prescribed drugs were worse than the original problem. "We would have to give drugs to counteract previous drugs," she said, "and most drugs were just covering up symptoms."

But, again, disillusionment is only part of the story, in that it sets a quest in motion. Professionals, of course, must be convinced they are doing the best for their patients—just as parents must be convinced they are doing the best for their children—and at first they, too, are likely to question the unfamiliar system of scientific logic that homeopathy represents.

Rudolph Ballantine, M.D., who directs the Center for Holistic Medicine in New York City and who integrates homeopathy in his practice, wrote in his book, *Radical Healing,* "I was hard put to believe there was anything to [homeopathy] myself. After I began practicing homeopathy and prescribing remedies to my patients, I still clung to some skepticism—the residue, perhaps, of my allopathic medical training. When patients told me they got better from the remedies, I would ask, almost surprised, 'You did? Are you sure?'"[2] Ultimately, what changed Dr. Ballantine's mind was a powerful remedy his homeopathic instructor prescribed for him. Aha!

Chicken Soup and Beyond

I mention professionals here not only to draw a parallel between them and Medicine Moms, but also because it is important to remember that there are a growing number of medical professionals who are embracing the homeopathic approach (see Chapter 4 for a discussion of how to locate one).

I would not want this book to convey the impression that Medicine Moms should—or could—do it all on their own. Along with the process of becoming informed, and learning about self-treatment for minor matters, seeking assistance and guidance from a trained professional is invaluable. Likewise, I would never suggest that Medicine Moms fail to make use of conventional medical interventions when they are warranted (more about this later as well). Conventional, or allopathic, medicine has its own remarkable achievements to boast of, and true Medicine Moms would not want to throw the baby out with the bath water.

On the other hand, *no one knows our families better than we do, and no one cares about their health like we do.* Imagine if you could combine your strong bond with your loved ones with a system of care that allows you to minister to them based on the very specific information you have about them and their needs. Imagine if you could empower yourself to help your family—and yourself—to reclaim a birthright of health and well-being. That is what this book aims to help you accomplish.

Chances are you already know more than you think you know about keeping your family well. Most moms do, and always have.

Were you ever given chicken soup by your own mother? ("Good for what ails you," she might have said.) Sure, it made you feel better because it was hot and tasty, and made with love. But when

researchers at Mount Sinai Medical Center in Miami Beach conducted randomized trials on flu sufferers using hot water, cold
water, and the proverbial chicken soup, the soup proved the most
effective liquid for clearing up nasal passages. It turns out an amino
acid plentiful in chicken is chemically similar to a drug prescribed
for bronchitis and other respiratory infections. What's more, in a
test tube experiment reported in the *New York Times,* chicken soup
inhibited the activity of certain white blood cells which caused in-
flammation that led to irritated airways and phlegm production.[3]

Chances are the vast majority of soup-pushing mothers knew
nothing about the broth's amino acid content or effect on white
blood cells. But they had sound instincts, and they saw what
worked. And that is common sense.

Robert S. Mendelsohn, M.D., in his wonderful book called *How
to Raise a Healthy Child . . . in Spite of Your Doctor,* affirmed that
"common sense is the most useful tool in dealing with illness."[4]
Alas, these days common sense in medical matters seems somewhat elusive, to say the least. Our culture has created many obsta-
cles to employing it. The next chapter examines some of the most
vexing ones.

CHAPTER

2

Beyond Good Guys and Bad Guys

The whole imposing edifice of modern medicine is like the celebrated tower of Pisa—slightly off balance.
—H.R.H. Prince Charles, quoted in the *London Observer*

The human immune system is a wondrous thing. While this book was being written, homage was paid it in an exhibit at New York City's Museum of Natural History, and I coaxed my family into attending.

We walked through a series of darkened rooms adorned with vastly enlarged and brightly colored replicas of microbes in the form of globes, spirals, and so many other sundry shapes they brought to mind a well-stocked pasta emporium. These rooms were meant to mimic the inner environment of the human body, which is in fact a habitat housing millions of microbes—many of which are harmless, some of which are helpful, and some of which are potentially dangerous pathogens.

The exhibit, which was entitled "Epidemic," was in large part a powerful reminder of the awesome vigilance and efficiency of the immune system in combating disease-causing bacteria, viruses, molds, yeasts, worms, and the like. Though many aspects of immunity and epidemiology were addressed, most of the exhibit's crowd-pleasing displays featured a "good guy versus bad guy"—immune system versus germs—motif. For instance one could, for both amusement and edification, tread upon the shadow outline of a human being, and by stepping on any part of it, call up an image of the disease organisms that might inhabit that particular body part. Likewise, in an interactive game, two players—one taking the role of the immune system, the other an ill-intentioned germ—could attempt to outstrategize one another.

A good time was had by all. And the good guy/bad guy "search and destroy" view of human immunity—in which enemy microbes are detected, engulfed, and neutralized with tactics that would make General Schwarzkopf proud—is in no way inaccurate. But it's just not complete.

The complexity and intelligence of the immune system far exceeds any one-dimensional view.

Whole Immunity

In *The Lives of a Cell,* a National Book Award–winning collection of insightful essays on the miracles of biology, the late Dr. Lewis Thomas (whose posts had included the presidency of New York's Memorial Sloan Kettering Cancer Center and a professorship in Pediatric Research at the University of Minnesota), praised "the sheer power of the human organism." He noted that its "surest tendency is toward stability and balance."

"It is a distortion," wrote Thomas, "with something profoundly disloyal about it, to picture the human being as a teetering, fallible contraption, always needing watching and patching, always on the verge of flapping to pieces." Then he suggested we develop an improved education system concerning human health "with more curricular time or acknowledgment, and even celebration, of *the absolute marvel of good health that is the real lot of most of us, most of the time.*"[1]

Immunology is still a young science, so mysterious and profound that it was rightly described as "Talmudic" by Dr. Baruj Benacerraf, a Nobel Laureate and Harvard Medical School professor.[2] Much about our immune functions is still unknown, but one of the things that is known is that the immune system is more concerned with making peace than with making war.

Remember, as humans we share our bodies with countless numbers of invisible minuscule organisms. Many pose no threat, but some do. For example, even as you sit reading this passage, hundreds of viruses are lurking within you. Sounds scary (and gross, as my son would say), but chances are astronomically high that you will finish this chapter, have a nice bit of supper, go to bed, and waken in the same robust good health with which you likely began the day. Why? Because your immune system is not so much warrior as diplomat—highly skilled at the art of peaceful coexistence.

Every day—every moment, in fact—your immune system is distinguishing between friend and potential foe, reacting to each microorganism appropriately, and striving not to overreact. When negotiations are successful, the result, generally, is a happy symbiosis and a healthy balance of power.

Now I say this state of affairs is a "known" fact. And scientifically it is. But emotionally, we still prefer the hero/villain, white hat/black hat view of biology. As Dr. Thomas puts it, despite such insights, "We still think of human disease as the work of an organized, modernized kind of demonology, in which bacteria are the most visible and centrally placed of our adversaries . . . These are paranoid delusions on a societal scale, explainable in part by our need for enemies."[3]

By "we," Thomas refers to both laypersons and to the kinds of well-meaning but misguided physicians who opt for extraordinary measures to deal with ordinary and unremarkable blips on the body's radar screen—the runny nose, the stuffy ear—employing the equivalent of a cannon to eradicate an annoying little flea. Employing extreme, speedy measures gives us a sense of control. But it is a false sense.

Above and Beyond

Speaking of how badly we want a sense of control, and at what cost, there is yet another way in which we tend to underappreciate the brilliance of the immune system. In general, we as a culture persist in viewing human immunity *only* as good cells using biological artillery to target bad ones—all on a simple mechanical level. The mechanical is part of the overall picture, to be sure. But the more we know about our own defense mechanisms, the more it becomes clear how much we don't know—or don't want to know.

For instance, it took us many years to begin to understand the negative effect of stress and the positive effects of emotional calm on the immune system. And some people continue to pooh-pooh that even though it is plainly demonstrable. (Stress levels raise adrenaline, steroids, and blood pressure in an attempt to direct the body's energy toward the "fight or flight" response. In this process, the entire body is pumped up except for the immune system, which becomes understaffed and inefficient.)

Now what about things that are not as easily explained by cause-and-effect, but are unarguably highly significant?

What, for example, are we to make of the countless people throughout human history whose medical conditions have markedly improved after being treated by a faith healer or tribal shaman (perhaps what we might call a "witch doctor")? What are we to make of the fact that clinical trials of new drugs which are invariably tested against a placebo (a plain sugar pill with no known physical medicinal effect) virtually always show that some subjects improve simply by taking the placebo? And what in the name of heaven are we to make of studies showing that prayer has a positive impact on healing?[4]

The truth is we aren't sure what to make of all this. But if we really consider all the evidence, it's plain we don't comprehend a fraction of what there is to know about the immune system. Certain of its aspects seem to function on intangible levels far beyond what our science is thus far even capable of comprehending.

Of course, I appreciate that this sounds a bit strange and mysterious. It flies in the face of our complacent assumption that modern medical science has all the answers, and all the answers are explainable. So why bring it up? Precisely to show how unsettling this sort of information can be. All of this mystery *could* be cause for rejoicing, and for celebrating the majesty and wisdom of our bodies and the vital forces that sustain them. But usually, it's not so joy-inducing. Usually it just frightens people into doing—or overdoing—the familiar.

Unfortunately, what is familiar is to underestimate our natural healing abilities and rely instead on those aforementioned flea-killing cannons—in other words, on pharmaceuticals, such as antibiotics.

What's Wrong with This Picture

There's no arguing the potential benefits of some antibiotics in some situations. Since their inception, antibiotics have saved countless lives. Would I endorse the use of antibiotics if a member of my family were faced with a serious health condition that warranted them over all other interventions? Would other Medicine Moms? You bet.

But are these drugs warranted as much as they're prescribed? Or do we tend to do too much because we are too frightened to leave well enough alone? Let me have the prestigious and unarguably mainstream *Journal of the American Medical Association* answer that one.

In its June 3, 1998 issue, *JAMA* reported on the treatment of acute otitis media (middle ear infection) in children. Among the contentions of the authors of two articles appearing in this issue are, first, that "too often, acute otitis media (AOM) is over-diagnosed" (physicians believe an infection exists where none does in 40 percent to 80 percent of all patients).[5] Second, even when infection exists, the condition can be as likely to clear up spontaneously as it is with antibiotics (recent evidence suggests that long-term outcomes in developed countries are similar in antibiotic-treated children and untreated children with AOM).[6]

What does this mean for you when, say, you take your child, who is suffering from a cold and mild fever, to the pediatrician? Most likely it means—again I quote *JAMA*—"the temptation is great to see a little bit of redness or fluid behind the eardrum as justification for antibiotic prescription."[7] Now, remember, chances are high this diagnosis might be wrong, and the ear redness could be caused by upset and crying, or fever, or even an allergic reaction. Or perhaps an ear infection is present but caused by a virus (against which antibiotics are ineffective) as opposed to bacteria. If so, the antibiotic your child is prescribed will prove useless. What's more, even if your child has an actual bacterial ear infection, the drug may well be superfluous.

But despite study after study that has been published or cited not only in *JAMA* but in numerous other mainstream medical journals (e.g., *Lancet, Canadian Family Physician, Archives of Otolaryngology*) which point to the fact that antibiotics are likely unnecessary in this typical scenario, many physicians are in a rut. *They are in the habit of underestimating what our bodies can do all by themselves.*

Hippocrates, the Greek physician generally acknowledged to be the father of contemporary medicine and whose Hippocratic oath physicians still take today, believed that the body has a natural tendency to heal itself. But today the body's innate wisdom is too often discounted. Most prescription drug-loyal doctors sincerely think they are doing the right thing in helping our immune systems along. They take a kind of Desert Storm approach to such a minor matter as an (alleged) ear infection, and send in what they perceive as the pharmaceutical equivalent of a "smart bomb" to target and eradicate "enemy" legions.

But as many of us parents have witnessed firsthand, such heroic measures are all too often a starting nudge down a slippery slope.

Antibiotics use can itself lead to all manner of problems that are iatrogenic—i.e., caused by the alleged "cure." They change the balance of intestinal flora (killing off the helpful bacteria) and can lead to intestinal tract problems such as diarrhea.[8] They can cause sensitivities and allergies, sometimes severe ones. My friend's one-year-old spent last Christmas day in the emergency room because his pediatrician had prescribed an antibiotic containing penicillin for an ear infection, not knowing the child would prove allergic to penicillin. (Ultimately, this provided an incentive for this mother's conversion to Medicine Momhood.)

If antibiotics don't clear up an infection or prevent its recurrence (which is all too often the case), they may inspire other medically invasive procedures such as the insertion of tubes in a child's ears, which is often recommended after several courses of antibiotics have failed to clear up AOM. This procedure is not without its own risks, including scarring, hardening of the eardrum with resulting hearing loss, infection from contaminants entering through the tube, and of course, the dangers posed by any procedure requiring a general anaesthetic. (And perhaps by now it will not surprise you to learn that controlled studies have shown that when both ears are infected and a tube is inserted in only one, the outcome for both ears is—you guessed it—identical.[9])

But beyond all this lies the most significant and frightening danger of antibiotics, one that potentially affects not just our kids, not just our families, but all of humanity. And this is no exaggeration. For when we dismiss and discount the body's innate healing powers and send in that proverbial cannon to slaughter a flea, some of the flea's aunts and uncles and cousins only get stronger and stronger as a result.

It's More Than Personal

In a cover story in May 1999, *U.S. News & World Report* proclaimed that we humans are, as the story's title put it, "Losing the Battle of the Bugs." It stated: "The rampant inappropriate use of [antibiotics] for colds and other ailments is contributing to the rise of resistant bacterial strains that cannot be treated. As many as half of outpatient antibiotic prescriptions a year are written unnecessarily, according to the Federal Centers for Disease Control and Prevention."[10]

This alarming story—and many similar ones which have appeared subsequently—explains how, ironically and tragically, antibiotics are perpetuating, and indeed worsening, the very problem they were meant to solve. The way this happens is not complicated: Drugs are sent in to kill the "bad guys," and manage to target many of them. But the most ornery of the "bad guys" (i.e. those bacteria that are genetically endowed with resistance to one or more antibiotics) remain standing. Through the process of natural selection, the survivors breed more of their own kind, and the cycle worsens. The immune system, which is naturally meant to create and thrive on a balance of power, is thrown way out of whack.

This presents a serious problem, and not just for the unfortunate patient who has taken too many courses of antibiotics when none were called for. It affects every one of us on the planet. Because bacteria are becoming, in effect, more and more potent, graver and graver health dangers exist. Should we legitimately need antibiotics to combat a life-and-death biological threat, there is a chance the drugs we swallow will, in effect, shoot blanks. This means, simply enough, your kids—even if they've never had a course of antibiotics in their lives—are at risk if their friends, neighbors, and schoolmates are persisting in taking too many. (And suburban families with kids are the nation's heaviest users of antibiotics![11])

If this sounds like science run amok—well, it's because that's just what it is. And that's what makes the Centers for Disease Control's contention that 50 percent of antibiotics are prescribed unnecessarily especially discouraging.

Since the inception of antibiotics in the 1940s, it's been observed that the more one is used, the quicker it becomes useless. Nowadays, antibiotic overuse is well publicized to medical professionals. Consumer watchdog groups are also promoting awareness of the problem. And one need only read the "precautions" accompanying any antibiotic to see for oneself such phrases as "prolonged administrations may result in overgrowth of nonsusceptible organisms." Yet, on many practitioners go, prescribing big-gun drugs for minor ailments.

A case in point is the friend I mentioned, whose child ended up in the hospital emergency room because of a reaction to a drug for an ear infection. A month or so later, this mom balked when her baby's pediatrician said, "Hmm, your baby has a little bit of fluid behind his ears. I'm going to prescribe an antibiotic for him to take for the next six weeks . . .

(Yes, he said six weeks!)

"Then," he continued, "there'll be a seventy-five percent chance that he won't develop an ear infection."

My friend was already a bit skeptical about the benefits of antibiotics when weighed against the risks. Now she balked. "I'm not Madame Curie," she said to me, "but this seemed to make no sense whatsoever."

Certainly it didn't. As three highly respected physicians—including the Chief of Infectious Diseases at Children's Hospital in Philadelphia—write in their book, *Breaking the Antibiotic Habit,* ear fluid alone is not a sign of bacterial infection, and only rarely will one develop. Children who receive antibiotics for this condition fare the same, if examined one month later, as those who don't.[12]

And so, despite the fact that my friend's prescription remained in her handbag, she returned to the pediatrician six weeks later to hear him say the baby's ears were totally clear. He was happy about how well the antibiotic worked(!) But the truth was something else again. Score one for the body's on-the-job skills.

Was this overzealousness to prescribe antibiotics an isolated incident? Clearly, and sadly, not. Indeed, as this book goes to press, 30 million annual prescriptions are being written to treat 10 million annual cases of middle ear infection.[13] That's *three prescriptions per case.*

But we can't just point fingers at doctors. It would solve nothing, and more to the point, it would ignore the complex web of reasons that have contributed to the health pickle in which we all find ourselves. Becoming a Medicine Mom is not about blaming, but healing. Since the best kind of healing requires understanding and compassion, let's start by having some for today's physicians, who find themselves in a tough spot.

Between a Rock, a Hard Place, and a Boulder

Let's imagine a hypothetical pediatrician. We'll call him Dr. White, for the "white hat" he likes to wear when fighting germs. Dr. White has been trained to make interventions—to *do something* when a patient comes to see him. He is, in the words of Melvin Konner, M.D., whose book *Becoming a Doctor* sheds light on the medical education process, an artisan. That means he is a highly skilled and specialized craftsman who sees his job as doing what any other doctor would do given similar circumstances. So he will prescribe an antibiotic, in part because he sincerely believes this is the most skillful service he can provide.

He will likely prescribe that antibiotic quickly (given the rate of misdiagnosis, sometimes too quickly). And that may be in part because that is what health insurance companies—who call the shots when it comes to the economics of his practice—will expect and reward.

He may also prescribe that antibiotic in an attempt to protect not only his patient, as he sees it, but himself—lest he later be sued for malpractice for *not* having prescribed one. As Konner writes, "In the norm there is safety. This is true in the ultimate legal sense: a judge will rule on alleged error or negligence contingent on the local standard of practice. If you do what is commonly accepted, not in medical journals or in the leading hospitals but in your local medical community, then you are probably safe."[14]

Moreover, the doctor would prescribe that antibiotic secure in the knowledge that drug companies have a strategy for combating the rampant drug overuse problem—which is to keep coming up with stronger and stronger drugs. (Which, yes indeed, lead to more and more hale and hearty resistant bugs, but their promotional campaigns don't dwell on that.)

Now, here's the real rub. Perhaps most of all, Dr. White might well prescribe that antibiotic *because that is what he thinks we want!* In a study of over 600 pediatricians, a whopping 96 percent of doctors surveyed reported that parents had recently requested antibiotics for their children when they were not indicated. One-third of the doctors admitted to complying with parents' demands.[15]

So, ironically enough—despite the doctors, the lawyers, the drug company sales reps, the HMO administrators, and whomever and whatever else you want to throw into the mix—it really does, in large measure, come right back down to us parents.

What Is Normal?

Now, just why would a parent insist on a prescription drug for her child, especially if the child's ailment was mild and unremarkable? The cynical answer, which I have on occasion encountered, is, "Well, they just want to hurry up and get back to their jobs." But I don't believe that is the case. I believe parents want what's best for their kids the way physicians want what's best for their patients—but we can all be woefully off the mark as to what the best is.

In America, we live in a "fix it" culture. Columnist Bill Bryson, who compared life in Britain and the United States in his book, *I'm a Stranger Here Myself,* contrasted the two countries' ways of thinking. "An advertisement in Britain for a cold relief capsule, for instance, would promise no more than that it might make you feel a little better . . . A commercial for the selfsame product in America, however, would guarantee total instantaneous relief." The author adds, "A person on the American side of the Atlantic who took this miracle compound would . . . feel better than he had in years."

That about sums it up. We want a magic bullet, and we want it now.

Add to this our strong psychic need to identify "enemies" and stomp out problems and you begin to spot a trend. We don't just want our doctors to help us battle bad guy bugs; we want to annihilate our germ "foes" on all fronts. Hence, the consumer craze for antibacterial lotions, potions, creams, cleaners, wet wipes, and the like (which researchers speculate may themselves speed up the growth of resistant bacterial strains) in lieu of good old-fashioned soap and water hygiene.

Now add to this our genuine desire to alleviate the discomforts of our offspring. We want to eradicate their symptoms at all costs, because we don't like to see our kids suffer—and because we find symptoms themselves unnerving. (As we'll soon see. the homeopathic approach views symptoms more realistically as immune system responses meant to help the body maintain balance.) But being short-term outlook kinds of folks, we don't stop to consider the long-term dangers of continually suppressing symptoms.

Such "suppress the symptoms at all costs" attitudes extend beyond the realm of antibiotics themselves to include other all too-common kinds of medications, such as the nebulizers and inhalants used to treat allergies, asthma, and the like.

Do you recall my neighbor Corrine, whose son was freed, via homeopathy, from the tyranny of his "machine"? When she went to register him for kindergarten, she was asked by the school nurse if little Pete had any medical conditions. Corrine replied he'd had reactive airway disorder but that it was successfully being treated homeopathically. The nurse, who had encountered some other Medicine Moms, was not shocked, but she was dubious. She assured my neighbor that if there ever was a problem, the school had a closet full of nebulizers on hand, and she added with pride that the Parents Association had just donated two portable machines to take along on field trips.

Now I ask you, is it normal that many of our children cannot seem to breathe properly without the assistance of mechanical paraphernalia? Is it normal for them to inhale substances whose small print precautions include potential side effects such as hypertension and "paradoxical bronchiospasms" that can be life threatening?

It may be an exaggeration to say we see it as normal. But far too many of us see it as routine. How on earth did we become so inured to this sort of thing?

Here we need to look at yet another characteristic of our culture, which is our desire to delegate to others responsibility for the physical well-being of our children and ourselves. Sure, many a parent may speak up and request such-and-such a drug from a doctor—perhaps specifically by name, as we are increasingly urged to do by advertisements for prescription medications. And maybe that makes us feel like we're in control. But really we'd like the buck to stop with someone else.

The very terminology we use when we speak of health matters affirms this desire. We call our physicians *health care providers,* part of a *health care delivery system.* We look to HMOs for *health maintenance.*

What if we were to assign more responsibility to ourselves? What if we were to take the common sense so valuable in fostering good health and add to it a true respect for the way our awe-inspiring immune systems were meant to function? And what if we were to find a form of medicine that not only doesn't discount these things, but actually incorporates them at its very heart?

The good news: It's already in existence. And all you need do is discover it for yourself.

CHAPTER 3

Homeopathy: What's Right with This Picture?

It is vain to do with more what can be done with less.
  —William of Occam, *Occam's Razor*

I will examine my close surroundings, where there must be means which have never been dreamed of, just because they were too simple . . .
  —Samuel Hahnemann
  Studies of Homeopathic Medicine

In his memoir on working for the Clinton administration, George Stephanopoulos recounts a remarkable anecdote. Once, he says, when he was "fluey from fatigue" from working on health care initiatives, the First Lady sent him a pick-me-up. It was "a carton of homeopathic cures accompanied by a note: 'We need to keep you healthy for health care!' H."[1]

Whether Hillary Clinton is a serious devotee of homeopathy or if this was simply a thoughtful gesture, I can't say. But whether she meant it to or not, her gift and note pointed out a fundamental difference between traditional "health care" and homeopathy. The former treats illnesses. The latter treats people—and aims to restore the state of good health and the balance it regards as the norm.

A Bit of History

Homeopathy is not a new phenomenon, and it is anything but a New Age contrivance. A distinguished empirical science, it was formally developed nearly two hundred years ago by German physician and pharmacist Samuel Hahnemann. I say *formally,* because although Hahnemann systematized homeopathy, some of its key principles were noted centuries earlier by both the Greeks and Renaissance philosophers, as well as in ancient Chinese and Indian medical texts, which like homeopathy expressed belief in the body's guiding intelligence.

At the time Hahnemann received his medical degree in 1779,

European medicine was in an especially bad way, with few effective therapeutic methods available. Physicians were still bleeding people with leeches, and drawing out what they referred to as "bad humors." His disenchantment was strong, and became greater still when his own daughter nearly perished at the hands of a conventional physician. Hahnemann resigned his practice to write and do research in the fields of chemistry, pharmacology, and toxicology, but in the course of his studies he was to stumble upon one of those "aha" experiences that usher in new ways of looking at the world.

Hahnemann had become intrigued with Hippocrates' thoughts on curing with similars—i.e. with substances that create symptoms akin to those of a given illness. With this in mind, he began experimenting with Chinchina bark from a Peruvian tree (the source of quinine), noting that if this substance was given to a healthy person, it produced symptoms similar to those of malaria. Through his continued research experiments—called "provings"—with healthy subjects, Hahnemann was to derive effective treatments for many of the ravaging epidemics of the nineteenth century, including cholera, typhoid, and yellow and scarlet fever.

For a dozen years Hahnemann pursued his studies, refining homeopathy's principles—among them, the use of smaller and smaller doses of curative substances. In 1796, he resumed medical practice, and in 1810 he published his first edition of his classic work, *The Organon of the Rational Art of Healing* (of which many subsequent editions were to follow). Due to its success in fighting infectious diseases, homeopathy achieved widespread popularity and credibility.

But you might wonder: If it was so popular and effective, why did it fall from favor? Actually, in much of the world it never has. Although allopathy, i.e. what we now think of as conventional Western medicine, was to take many great leaps forward in ensuing years, homeopathy has remained a prominent form of medicine in England, France, Germany, and Belgium, as well as in India and parts of Latin America. In the United States, homeopathy also gained a strong foothold. At the turn of the century America had some 12,000 homeopathic physicians and 22 homeopathic hospitals. However, sociopolitical forces were such that this system of medicine was effectively squelched by its competitors.[2]

Today's resurgence of interest is due, quite simply, to consumer demand. And consumer demand is present because homeopathy—as forged by Hahnemann and elaborated upon by thousands of practitioners around the world for two centuries—works.

Now for some avid consumers the mere fact that homeopathy works is all they want to know. They may swear by homeopathy, but they don't exactly know what it is. There's nothing wrong with that position. My car works very nicely, thank you, but I couldn't give a fig how it conveys me to the supermarket or the train station.

Yet the more involved with homeopathy many of us become, the more naturally curious we grow about its guiding principles. For those of you in this category, as well as for the many of you who may not yet be involved with homeopathy but would like more information before venturing to try it, the remainder of this chapter is devoted to explaining some of its underlying tenets.

The Law of Similars

You may recall the story I told about how astonished my neighbor was when a homeopathic dose of *Allium cepa* (red onion) rapidly relieved her allergy-induced runny nose and teary eyes. What she was experiencing was the Law of Similars at work. First posited by Hippocrates in the fifth century B.C. and resurrected by Hahnemann and his followers, *Simila similibus curantur* ("Like shall be cured by like") is the cornerstone of homeopathy.

In homeopathic treatment, when a natural substance in a large dose tends to cause a particular symptom in a healthy individual—

the way red onion would cause tearing—that same substance, in a small dose, is used to stimulate the recovery of an ill person suffering from a like symptom. Thus, where a large dose of Ipecac would induce vomiting, a tiny homeopathic dose becomes one of the homeopathic remedies for nausea and vomiting. Where a large dose of *belladonna* causes flushing, someone whose fever is accompanied by flushed face may be a good candidate for a homeopathic dose of *belladonna,* which would help the body heal itself.

On an intuitive level, this may ring a bell with you. For although you are unlikely to hear the principle of *Simila similibus curantur* batted around today, we do have a phrase that roughly correlates. "Hair of the dog that bit him," we say. Likes are cured by likes.

In its tendency to treat a disturbance by moving ever so slightly in the same direction as that disturbance, and not oppositionally, homeopathy is the martial art of medicine. If you've ever studied or watched jujitsu, karate, and so on, you know what I mean. If an opponent is on the attack, what would you do to resist? Use the force of the attacker himself as your defense! Likewise, what are you told to do when you are driving, hit a slippery patch of roadway, and skid? Steer into the skid! If you try to fight it, you will likely crash.

Again, all of this may seem intuitive. But conventional Western medicine does not, in general, subscribe to the Law of Similars philosophy. There are some exceptions to be sure—for example, allergy shots are made from allergens—but much of traditional Western medicine could be viewed not as *like cures like* but as *contrary cures contrary.* That's why we have so many *anti*histamines, *anti*inflammatories, *anti*febriles, *anti*biotics, and the lot. Do these medications reverse symptoms? Obviously, in many cases they do. But in many instances the problem is backlash, especially if they are *over*used. What happens if you take too many laxatives? Constipation. What happens if you overdo nasal spray? A perennially clogged nose.

In homeopathy, this sort of backlash problem is anything but typical, especially if one obeys its second fundamental tenet—the Law of the Minimum Dose.

The Law of the Minimum Dose

Through careful experiments by Hahnemann and other early homeopaths, it was discovered that while large doses of "similars" would often evoke healing, there could be numerous side effects. In an attempt to minimize these, smaller and smaller amounts of medicinal substances were used. Amazingly, it was discovered that infinitesimal doses could have extremely beneficial actions, while side effects diminished correspondingly.

Just how small are typical homeopathic doses?

Very small.

Take, for example, a bottle of *Allium cepa* labeled with a "potency" of 6C (a typical potency you would find in your drugstore or health food store). That would mean one part red onion was soaked in alcohol and mixed with 99 parts water. The mixture was then vigorously shaken (or "succussed," as homeopathic terminology goes), then one part of *that* mixture was mixed with 99 parts water—again— and shaken. In all, the process was repeated six times, yielding 6C.

You see, I told you it is a very, very small dose. And homeopathy even goes on from there. For a 12C potency, the process would have been repeated a dozen times.

Now, with a potency above 12C things become downright confounding. According to a mathematical constant known as Avogadro's number, once you get past the 12C dilution level, there would not be one molecule of the original substance remaining intact. However, taking potencies above 12C is by no means uncommon.

This, of course, defies conventional logic. The truth is that no one—including even medical doctors who swear by homeopathy's effectiveness—quite understands the precise physical mechanism of homeopathic healing. Fascinating theories, however, abound.

Most of these theories have to do with the release of energy that occurs during each stage of dilution and succussion, and the "imprint" or "signature" that the original substance leaves on water molecules themselves. The hypotheses often involve advanced concepts in such things as quantum physics, chaos theory, wave function, hydrogen bonds, holography, and the like—and incite studies with names like *The Effect of Highly Diluted Agitated Thyroxine on the Climbing Activity of Frogs.*[3] You will more than likely be pleased that I am not going to try to attempt to expound on these theories here (though I refer you to the References and the Resources sections at the back of this book, if you're inclined to learn more).

For now, suffice it to say that at the heart of homeopathy is a mystery that many believe will be unraveled in the not too distant future as the sciences of physics and chemistry continue to progress. But again, the most important thing about homeopathy is not *how* it works but *that* it works.

Where's the Proof?

Work, it does. And the evidence goes far beyond the anecdotal.

At this point, numerous high-quality studies have been conducted on homeopathic medications, and overwhelmingly their findings support homeopathy's clinical effectiveness. They can't all be listed here, of course, but these are some examples, as reported in mainstream medical journals:

- Reported in *Biomedical Therapy:* In a study of 131 children, parents were allowed to choose homeopathic or conventional treatment for ear infection (acute otitis media). The total recurrences of the group treated homeopathically were far fewer than the group treated with antibiotics.[4]
- Reported in *Pediatrics:* In a study comparing individualized high-potency homeopathic preparations against a placebo in 81 children suffering from acute diarrhea, the homeopathic treatment group benefited from a statistically significant speed of recovery.[5]
- Reported in *Lancet:* In a double-blind study (where neither

patient nor researcher knows who is being treated with placebo or medication), 144 patients with active hay fever were given either a placebo or a high-dilution homeopathic preparation of grass pollens. The patients using homeopathy showed greater improvement in symptoms.[6]

• Reported in *Lancet:* In another double-blind, placebo-controlled study—this one with asthmatic patients—conducted at Europe's largest medical school, the University of Glasgow, researchers found that 80 percent of the patients given a homeopathic remedy improved, as opposed to 38 percent of those given a placebo. The patients were assessed by both a homeopathic and a conventional doctor. Moreover, the outcome of homeopathic asthma treatment studies were shown by the researchers to be reproducible.[7]

Certainly it may be argued that any one study can be erroneous or misleading. But precisely for this reason researchers have, of late, conducted thorough meta-analyses of homeopathic studies. In other words, they thoroughly reviewed the data contained in numerous studies that already have been done.

In one such meta-analysis, published in *Lancet,* a review of 186 studies revealed that patients taking homeopathic medicines were 2.45 times more likely to experience positive therapeutic effects than those taking placebo.[8] In another widely cited study, published in the *British Medical Journal,* 107 studies were reviewed, and 77 percent of those showed positive outcomes for homeopathic medicines.[9] The researchers, dubious, reduced the number of studies to only the most rigorous, i.e. the ones with the most thorough criteria and careful procedures. Homeopathy passed their scrutiny with flying colors. Of the 22 best studies, 15 showed the efficacy of homeopathy. The researchers concluded that, "The evidence presented in this review would probably be sufficient for establishing homeopathy as a regular treatment for certain indications." They added that the positive findings among the best studies "came as a surprise."

How often homeopathy surprises even the most skeptical!

Are You Sure It's Not just the Placebo Response?

As you can see, many of these studies show that homeopathy is more than a placebo response. That is, people are not getting better solely because they believe they will. Before I located these studies, I had informally and unwittingly confirmed this in my own household, as have many other Medicine Moms.

When I gave homeopathic *chamomilla* tablets to my teething infant, he most certainly did not expect that the tiny tabs melting on his tongue would make him feel any better. Yet they did. When I took a page from veterinary homeopathy and put a dose of *arnica*—for physical trauma and bruising—in my cat's water bowl after her oral surgery, she perked right up and began chewing her food, although I had been told this would not happen for another twenty-four to forty-eight hours. In my prejudiced view, of course, my cat is brighter than your average beast, but trust me, she was clueless as to my medicinal intervention and to the contents of her water dish.

Yet having said all this, it's only fair to note that the placebo response can, under the right circumstances, factor in virtually any kind of medical treatment. Some of the subjects given placebos in the aforementioned clinical trials *did* improve, even though a greater number improved on homeopathy, and as we already know, some patients invariably get better during studies of new prescription drugs which are also routinely tested against placebos.

What's going on? Surely the placebo, which is merely an inert sugar pill, itself does nothing. But the placebo *effect*—the thoughts and feelings attached to the taking of that little pill—is something else entirely. No one exactly knows the "how" of the placebo effect (yet another mystery to ponder), but we more or less can explain the "why." It works because mind and body are linked, and because mental expectations can influence physical outcome.

The placebo effect can incorporate many variables—a positive attitude, a compliant patient (who wants to get better to "please" the doctor), belief in the power of medications taken, faith in the skills of the physician. Somehow, one or more of these variables can initiate a self-healing response. Now here's where homeopathy has yet another advantage.

When one visits a homeopath, the rapport developed between patient and practitioner is likely to be very different from the one that is developed during a visit to a conventional doctor. It has been proven that there is more to homeopathy than belief, but since belief can play a role in any cure, let's see how and why homeopathy inspires it.

Beyond "Open Your Mouth and Say 'Ahh . . .' "

On a typical visit to the doctor, we are administered to by a practitioner in a white coat. According to a study by our now familiar friends at the *Journal of the American Medical Association,* the doctor will spend, on average, 23.1 seconds listening to our presenting complaint before interrupting us.[10] Soon after, if it's determined we have a treatable symptom, it's likely that inscrutable but authoritative scribbles will be made on a prescription pad. Granted, some people experience a placebo effect from what they perceive as the clinical, businesslike nature of this encounter, and unconsciously begin self-healing as a result. But consider the likelihood of this happening versus the potential in a typical visit to a homeopath.

According to another AMA journal, the *Archives of Family Medicine,* homeopathic physicians spend more time with their patients than their conventional counterparts.[11] They also order fewer tests, says the study, and prescribe fewer pharmaceutical medications. So just what is it that they do?

I'll let my neighbor Corrine answer, by recounting what happened when she first took her son to a homeopath:

When I called to make the appointment, I was told I'd be sent a questionnaire to fill out ahead of time, which would essentially

*help me to "write a story" about my son and his ailments. I
couldn't believe how much came out in the process. It took me
four legal-size pages to write everything that had happened to
Pete as we'd tried one treatment after another for his respiratory problems. When we gave it to the doctor, he reviewed it.
Then he spent a long time talking to Pete. Of course, he wanted
to hear what his congestion sounded like, but it seemed like he
also wanted to get to know Pete, and see how he felt about his
cough. All the others wanted to have a quick look-see and pull
out the prescription pad. We might spend an hour in a waiting
room, but then we were always in and out of the doctor's pres-
ence in a flash. Sometimes I'd be told, "Well, this drug is new—
let's try it." I felt like my child was a guinea pig. With
homeopathic treatment, I knew the doctor had a sense of
exactly who my son was.*

Corrine and Pete spent about forty-five minutes with the homeopathic physician, which is not unusual for a first consultation.
(Their typical "well visit" to their pediatrician took ten minutes.) At
the end, they both felt they had been taken seriously. Under-
standably, this sort of encounter could conceivably result in the be-
ginnings of self-healing, which might well aid any homeopathic
remedies taken. And if it does, that doesn't negate homeopathy's
clinical effectiveness. It only enhances it.

Why Are Homeopaths So Nosy?

Please don't misunderstand. The main purpose of a homeopath's
extensive quest for information about the patient is not to initiate a
placebo response. This may or may not be a wonderful side benefit
of the homeopathic fact-finding method. The thoroughness of a
homeopath is about finding out what—precisely and in what way—
is ailing the patient.

Homeopaths view symptoms with curiosity, even respect. To a

conventional physician, a symptom is often viewed as something to be conquered. Moreover, a group of symptoms may be viewed as unrelated problems, each one to be "corrected" individually. From a homeopathic perspective, symptoms are viewed as the body's attempt to heal itself. They tell a story, "speaking" of what is out of balance in the body. And oftentimes no matter how disparate symptoms may appear to be, they are part of the same underlying story. As Hahnemann put it in *The Organon,* "A single symptom is no more the whole disease than a single foot a whole man."

When you bring your child to a homeopath—or visit one for yourself—you will doubtless answer a goodly number of questions. Not surprisingly, he'll want to know about family history, previous traumas, surgical procedures, and so on, and he will also pose such common queries as:

- What is the chief complaint?
- When did it begin?
- What symptoms go along with the complaint?

But then he'll likely ask some deeper questions, such as:

- What else was happening in your life around the time this complaint started?
- What makes the symptoms more or less severe?
- Is there a time of day when the symptoms are worst?

Finally, he'll want to know a number of general things about the patient which relate to constitutional traits, temperament, and character, such as:

- What kind of weather does the patient prefer?
- Does he tend to be a "hot person" or a "chilly person?"
- What kinds of foods does he crave?
- What position does she sleep in?
- Does he have recurrent dreams?

- Does she weep when scolded?
- Is he tidy or messy?
- Is she self-confident? Sympathetic? Stubborn?
- How does he deal with frustration or disappointment?
- What music does he like, and how does it affect him?

Why does the homeopath want to know so much? And why does he seem so attentive and observant? Is he a nice, friendly guy? Well, he might be, but that's not what guides him in practice. Is he a busybody? Well, only because he has to be.

Because he aims to treat a person—a one-of-a-kind individual—who has an illness, rather than the illness in and of itself, the homeopath needs to see the whole picture, comprehend the entire individual. An empirical scientist at heart, a detective in spirit, he knows that what's unique about a case can shed a great deal more light than what's common about it. And he is always in search of the seemingly inconsequential details that may make everything clear. The homeopath's ultimate goal is to find the most appropriate remedy, which will restore the patient to the natural harmony of good health.

Because homeopathic remedies are specifically tailored to individuals and their unique sets of circumstances, don't be shocked if you and your neighbor both take your children in for earaches and walk away from your consultations with two different remedies.

The homeopath knows that all earaches are not created equal (some, for example, are right-sided, some left-sided; some are accompanied by fever, and/or thirst, some not, and so on). Neither are all asthma episodes. The same homeopath would want to know if an episode was preceded by exposure to an allergen, or an emotional upset. This may sound odd, but think about it. When you have had colds, have they all felt the same, or followed the same course? Were someone to take the trouble to ask you about them, it's certain you could distinguish one from another in detail.

Another thing the "detective" homeopath will be looking to determine is if the complaint of the patient was formed in successive layers. Here's an example: Let's say your child was diagnosed with several ear infections, given antibiotics to no avail, had tubes inserted into his ears (and been emotionally upset by the procedure), then *did* stop contracting ear infections—only to come down with recurrent bouts of bronchitis. Now let's say you read somewhere that the remedy *phosphorus* is often prescribed for bronchitis. Will your homeopath recommend it for your child? Don't be surprised if he doesn't—if instead he says your child will need something to counter the impact of so many courses of antibiotics, and then perhaps something for the after-effects of emotional distress (either or both of which may have driven the original problem deeper into the body).

This may sound like a bigger to-do than you had in mind, but it's no reason to be discouraged. If a chronic condition was formed over much time, in successive layers, it often needs to be undone in the same way. But at each step along the path, the body's balance will be restored.

Once again this is because the symptoms are not the illness itself, but a roadmap to the overall system's weak points. It takes more than a microbe to make us ill. Remember, we are all exposed to them all the time. It takes an inability on our part to do what comes naturally and compensate for any problem. The homeopath seeks to enable us to go back to doing what we were meant to do in the first place. He does this by bolstering not just the mechanical aspects of the immune system but the entire vital force that sustains us.

As parents, we often feel that time is of the essence. We want our kids to feel better, and feel better right away. And heaven knows we all have busy lives and hectic schedules to maintain. Conventional medicine, therefore, can seem like the quickest means to an end. But as most of us know firsthand, a quick fix can often lead to a relapse—and at the expense of the body's overall health.

Sure, a course of homeopathic treatment may take longer than a course of antibiotics or other pharmaceuticals. But at its conclusion—and usually along the way to its conclusion—there is a tremendous benefit to general well-being. Don't be surprised if, once all your child's "layers" have been peeled back, they not only have had their immediate illness cleared up, but may also sleep better, eat better, have more energy, and perhaps have even a longer attention span.

Is homeopathy a cure-all or a panacea? I don't mean to imply that at all. But done correctly, it can be an astonishing experience.

Is Homeopathy the Same as "Herbal Medicine"?

At this point, there is a common confusion that ought to be cleared up. Medicines categorized as "alternative" often tend to be lumped together, sometimes even by people one hopes would know better—like members of the media who cover this subject, or even the occasional clerk at a pharmacy and health food store. Because of this, homeopathy and herbal medicine are often confused, and the terms may be used interchangeably. Yet there are, in fact, some important differences.

Herbs are drawn strictly from plant matter. Homeopathy draws remedies from virtually any substance that could, in extremely small quantities, serve as a curative remedy. Such substances do include plants, herbs, trees, flowers, and fungi, but also salts, minerals, shells, metals, and animal products (e.g., cuttlefish ink). I once heard a physician at a homeopathic conference joke that any substance could be turned into a remedy—"from flatus to moonbeams." And he wasn't far off.

In addition, homeopathic remedies tend to be extremely specific, whereas herbal remedies are broad. For instance, a patient who complains of depression to a homeopath might receive one of dozens of different remedies depending on her precise symptoms, which would be minutely detailed in consultation. On the other hand, if the same patient were to seek an herbal remedy for depression, she would most likely be given St. John's wort, period. That might work fine, but only if she fit the symptom profile on which St. John's wort works best.

More importantly, herbalism does not follow the Law of the Minimum Dose, nor the Law of Similars. Herbalists use plant matter in comparatively large doses, whether in teas, tinctures, extracts, or dried pill form. This may certainly achieve a desired effect—let's say cayenne pepper and garlic to bring on heat—but the effect tends to be more like that of conventional pharmaceuticals. It aims to counter a symptom with a substance that ushers in an opposing condition. This can be done to the point where it suppresses symptoms in the short term at the expense of long-term health. It can also cause unpleasant side effects or even dangerous consequences, such as allergic reactions, high blood pressure, and kidney and liver damage. Like conventional medicines, some herbs, such as natural laxatives, can even be habit forming and cause dependency.

Having said all that, I want to be clear: Herbal medicine can be a very effective healing system—especially useful in occasionally purging and cleansing the body—and more is being discovered about it all the time. I've taken herbs when appropriate, and on one occasion where the right homeopathic remedy proved elusive, my son was given herbs—with a happy result. The herbs were, however, given under the close supervision of a pediatrician who knows a good bit about the subject. She monitored the exact dosage based on my son's body weight, and also provided herbs of whose purity she could be certain.

I think it would be wonderful for Medicine Moms to learn about herbs. But homeopathy, in general, is a gentler and more benign system. As such, it's the ideal first line of defense against illness.

Kids Like "Magic Water"!

To top it all off, I've saved what many Medicine Moms consider the best for last. If you have ever had the experience of your child wincing or wailing pitifully when faced with yet another spoonful of gloopy antibiotic or even, as mine did, commenting "Ugh" at a glass of juice laced with a mix of bitter herbs, you will be delighted at little ones' reactions to homeopathic remedies.

The meltaway tablets or pellets that are impregnated with the remedy are typically made from milk sugar, and since the remedy itself is so diluted, the mildly sweet tablet is all the child tastes. Many remedies for infants, such as teething or colic remedies, are now manufactured in individual doses and encapsulated in disposable plastic droppers—so you just snap one open, pour its contents into your baby's mouth, and *voilà*. Or you can take a pellet, dilute it in water yourself, and offer a palatable spoonful.

My son and his friends got so used to taking medicine this way they gave it a name—"magic water." And we, their moms, adopted it. For we couldn't have said it any better if we'd tried.

CHAPTER

4

I Want To, but I'm Scared . . .

The skeptic does not mean he who doubts, but he who investigates or researches, as opposed to he who asserts and thinks that he has found.
　　　　　—Miguel de Unamuno, Spanish philosopher,
　　　　　　　　Essays and Soliloquies

"Skepticism," is that anything more than we used to mean when we said, "Well, what have we here?"
　　　　　　　　　　　　　　　—Robert Frost

Whenever I'm about to try something new and out of the ordinary, I can't help having some doubts and making some second guesses. This makes me totally typical. What helps me most is getting more information, and also feeling that I'm not alone—that other normal, intelligent people have reached similar conclusions and made similar choices.

Well, anyone considering using homeopathy is anything but alone. In many countries around the world, this system of medicine is a run-of-the-mill first line of defense against illness for millions upon millions of people.

In France, it is estimated that 32 percent of the general practitioners prescribe homeopathic medicines on a regular basis, as do many specialists, including pediatricians. At least 39 percent of the population uses homeopathy routinely, and 75 percent approve of homeopathy. Nearly all French pharmacies stock homeopathic remedies, and homeopathic medicines are reimbursed under the national health care.

In Germany, about 1.5 million people are treated homeopathically each year and there are about 3,000 homeopathic practitioners who have specialist training—which has been accepted by the German Federal Medicaid Council as an additional medical qualification.

England has four homeopathic hospitals and millions of advocates, including members of the royal family. Homeopathy is also widely used and accepted in Belgium, the Netherlands, and Italy. Likewise in Russia, India, and many parts of South America.

In America, homeopathy use, after a dormant period, is rising like a phoenix from the ashes. Since 1990, its growth has been estimated at 20 to 30 percent per year.[1] Along with other so-called "complementary and alternative therapies" (commonly known in the medical community by the acronym CAM), it is part of a popular groundswell that is only going to grow larger as the new millennium unfolds.

CAM Can

Interest in CAM can no longer even remotely be considered radical or "kooky" or even nonmainstream. It is interwoven in the fabric of American culture.

In a survey on alternative health trends published at the end of 1998 in the *Journal of the American Medical Association,* the conclusions reached were clear. Use of alternative therapies increased substantially in the United States between 1990 and 1997. (Homeopathy was listed as one of those increasing the most.) What's more, the increase was clearly due to more people choosing alternative treatments, as opposed to the already converted simply using them more often.[2]

The demand for alternative therapies is so strong, and interest running so high, that *JAMA* reports a majority of U.S. medical schools now offer courses in CAM. A good thing too, because most medical students say they want this as part of their curriculum.

Additionally, more and more pharmacists are reporting customer interest in alternative medicines. A quick look around your drugstore shelves will reveal many new successful products that incorporate homeopathic remedies (such as Coldeeze®, which uses zinc in a homeopathic potency), as well as many conventional products in new "natural" versions.

If all this isn't enough to make you feel CAM in general—and homeopathy in particular—has an "official" stamp of approval, consider this: The U.S. Army Breast Cancer Research Program has recommended funding a study examining the use of homeopathic medicines for hot flashes and other menopausal symptoms in a group of breast cancer survivors. The cost of the study: one quarter of a million dollars.[3] Yes, our tax dollars. What can be more official than that?

All in all, this adds up to far more than a whim or passing fancy. Enthusiasm about CAM is strong not because it is a trend. Just the opposite: CAM is a trend because we need it, and because we as a society have matured enough to begin to be able to accept it.

Getting Support

Still and all, if being a Medicine Mom today is to be part of a swelling movement, we are a vanguard nonetheless. Though the numbers tilting in our favor are impressive, there is resistance as well. One of the best ways to meet that resistance and bolster one's confidence—while continuing the quest for more and more valid information—is to make contact with like-minded people.

My own network of Medicine Moms got started informally, one might say accidentally on purpose. One person told another, who told another and so on. Soon we were all trading tips, advice, and resources. And wherever one of us went—be it to work, or to volunteer groups, or to the hairdresser's—we seemed, without quite planning on it, to add to our numbers. We became Johnny Appleseeds of homeopathy. In fact, when one of us relocated to another part of the state for a year for business reasons, she returned to us having created an ad hoc "branch" of our group many miles away.

Given the serendipitous way the universe seems to work, if you are nursing a serious hankering to be in touch with Medicine Moms, or would-be Medicine Moms, it may just happen—as it did to me—that you will meet some at exactly the right moment. But then again, don't be afraid to take a proactive stance and give the Fates a poke in the right direction.

This is easy to do by getting in touch with a wonderful nonprofit organization called the National Center for Homeopathy (see the Resources section on how to do this). NCH has a nationwide network of what are called Affiliated Study Groups whose members (usually interested laypersons) meet on a regular basis to learn about homeopathy and self-care. You may well find a group in your area that would be delighted to hear from you. If there is no group near you, you can refer to the annual member directory to locate individuals in your area with an interest in homeopathy.

Once you and a few others get together, however you find each other, you can, if you like, begin your own study group. There is a lot of useful support material, including a very helpful study guide, available from the NCH. Of course, if meeting regularly is not your style, or does not fit into your schedule, you may opt to form a loose sort of "daisy chain" of Medicine Moms whose encouragement and practical suggestions are only a phone call away.

Finding a Homeopath

Together with other Medicine Moms, you may want to test the waters, so to speak, by trying homeopathic remedies that are meant to treat routine self-limiting conditions—like teething pains, sunburn, minor bruises, or runny noses—that may affect you or your family members. It is always rewarding to share those amazing initial "Aha!" experiences with appreciative pals.

Still another reason it is wonderful to be in touch with other Medicine Moms is to get help in finding a homeopath. For serious medical conditions or for chronic complaints (i.e., conditions that have lasted for some weeks or months, or which keep recurring), it is eminently sensible to seek professional expertise.

Finding a medical professional that you like and trust, and to whom you have reasonable access, is always a challenging task, no matter what sort you are searching for. When it comes to finding a homeopath in particular, you should first familiarize yourself with who practices homeopathy.

Many M.D.s (medical doctors) and D.O.s (osteopathic doctors) study homeopathy as a postgraduate specialty; naturopathic physicians (N.D.s) study homeopathy as part of their routine school training. Members of both these groups may have board certification, consisting of a Diplomate in Homeotherapeutics (D.Ht.) for M.D.s and D.O.s, and a Diplomate of the Homeopathic Academy of Naturopathic Physicians (DHANP) for N.D.s.

Other professionals who sometimes practice homeopathy within the scope of their licensure include chiropractors, dentists, nurse-midwives, nurse practitioners, physician assistants, and—not to leave any of your family members untended to—veterinarians. Some of these may have earned a Certificate in Classical Homeopathy (CCH) from the Council for Homeopathic Certification, which publishes a directory of those who have passed its notoriously rigorous exam. (See the Resources section for their contact information.)

If all these initials and credentials leave you a bit befuddled, don't worry. As this book is being written, there are over two thousand conventionally trained American physicians who practice homeopathy, as well as some five thousand chiropractors, and three to five thousand nurses, dentists, and other assorted practitioners. And the best way to find those among them that suit your needs is to use the same tried-and-true strategy that works for finding anything: word of mouth!

If someone is going to dispense a critical service to my family, I want to know that they have successfully done the same for other people. Certainly I want them to have the appropriate credentials and experience, but I also want to know that they are trustworthy, that I can get them on the phone within a reasonable amount of time, that they won't talk down to me, and that they'll take my check. I also want to know if they seem to have some essential and intuitive "gift" or "flair" for what they do. (Some healers simply seem to have natural healing abilities, and when we meet them, we recognize them.) What's more, if they are going to be dealing with my kid, I want to know if they genuinely like kids, and if kids in turn like them.

Who better to tell me these things than other moms?

Of course, once you have your first appointment with a practitioner, you will be able to judge for yourself whether the "fit" is right for you and your family. And once they have had time to initiate treatment, your proof will be in the proverbial pudding. If things are improving, you're obviously on the right track. For as Paracelsus bluntly and perfectly put it, "He who heals is right."

Feel free to pass all kinds of information, positive and negative, along your Medicine Mom network. For soon you, too, will become a critical link in the chain.

Encountering Skeptics

Having support in the form of other Medicine Moms and/or a practitioner with a sound reputation should make you much more secure in your decision to try homeopathy. Realistically, however, your resolve and enthusiasm may from time to time be somewhat diluted by determined friends, acquaintances, and even family members who, having learned of your interest in homeopathy, will be dubious—perhaps even aghast. Dealing with this sort of encounter may be the most challenging part of your transition to Medicine Mom, but it also offers a great opportunity.

If you can explain your position calmly and factually, you won't sound defensive—and who knows, you may even be sowing the seeds of the future expansion of Medicine Momhood. But remember, the goal in dealing with a skeptic is neither to preach nor to pressure. Nor, for that matter, is it to bore. It is only to inform, *if* someone *wants* information.

With all this in mind, this next section is devoted to a series of *Questions and Answers*. The *Questions* are typical queries that skeptical inquisitors may ask once they learn of your new interest. They are perfectly legitimate questions, and indeed may be some of the ones you yourself posed—or are still wondering about—as you learn more about the practice of homeopathy.

The *Answers* are offered in two modes, which I term *The Long of It* and *The Short of It.* The long answers are detailed and useful, I hope, in coping with any lingering doubts of your own, as well as in replying to your conversation partner in the course of a full-fledged serious discussion (the kind where the person asking the question sincerely wants to hear the answers, and not just goad you). The short answers are abbreviated, slightly more deflective versions of the long ones. They should prove especially useful in situations or places where it's not appropriate or desirable to get into a long, drawn-out discussion (cocktail parties and T-ball bleachers come to mind), or when the person asking you questions is someone you suspect isn't really ready, willing, or able to assimilate detailed replies.

Instinctively, I'm sure you'll know just which to use when, or when you may need to switch from one mode to another in midstream. (Hint: if someone's eyes are glazing over, switch from a *Long Answer* to a *Short Answer.*) Please do remember, every question asked of you offers you an opportunity both to teach and to learn. That's why it's best never to begrudge anyone his or her right to ask.

Some Questions and Answers

Q. How can you just ignore conventional medicine, with all its obvious benefits?

The Long of It: The combination of conventional and alternative medicine is what results in the terms "complementary" or "integrative" medicine. One need not exclude the other. In fact, there are no known "drug interaction" problems with homeopathy. So you can take homeopathic remedies alongside allopathic medications when that seems to make sense. Sometimes so-called "alternative" remedies can bolster the immune system and negate or diminish the side effects of conventional drugs. This sort of strategy has proved very effective for countless people. Many with life-threatening illnesses, such as cancer, take complementary medications to mitigate the effects of chemotherapy, for example. Homeopathy also uses substances, such as the dilute remedy made from the *thuja* tree, that can counteract the harmful effects of antibiotics.

The Short of It: We're not. We do whatever works most effectively and does the least harm.

Q. Don't you realize how lucky we are to live in an age when antibiotics are available?

The Long of It: Yes, but living in an age when antibiotics are abused is akin to living in an age before they were discovered. That's because if they are used too much, these drugs will stop being effective when they need to be. There is no longer any question whatsoever that antibiotic overuse can lead to the evolution of highly resistant bacteria. The Centers for Disease Control, the American Academy of Pediatrics, and even the pharmaceutical firms warn against using antibiotics indiscriminately. Many developed countries, including Japan, Iceland, and Finland have launched national campaigns educating the public about the issue.

And who is at highest risk for being affected by highly resistant bacteria? Kids. Especially those under six, who live in the suburbs, with relatively affluent parents who take them to doctors frequently.[4] Sound like anyone you know?

The Short of It: Absolutely. We just don't like to overuse or abuse them. You can have too much of a good thing.

Q. What about the dangers of not treating an ear infection quickly, like hearing problems and delayed speech?

The Long of It: These are probably not as great as the dangers involved in rushing to treat an ear infection that may very well be caused by a virus (antibiotics would be useless for it anyhow) or that may not even be an infection at all. I'm not a doctor, so you may not believe me. Just read *Breaking the Antibiotics Habit* by Paul Offit. He's Chief of Infectious Diseases at Children's Hospital in Philadelphia, so he ought to know.

By the way, Dr. Offit points out that kids in Norway, Sweden, Denmark, and Holland are simply not given antibiotics for ear infections. And we haven't heard of any rampant speech or hearing deficits in those countries. I know plenty of people from my own generation who weren't given antibiotics for ear infections as kids, and they hear loud and clear.

The Short of It: I've been doing some reading, and perhaps those dangers are overstated. But I understand your caution. If you like, I can tell you how to get more information.

Q. Where are these homeopathic "remedies" made? In someone's kitchen?

The Long of It: In the very beginning, homeopaths had to produce their own medications, and sources were not always reliable. But this is far from the case today. Now the manufacture of homeopathic medicines is a big, international business. For example, the world's largest manufacturer, Boiron, sells some 3,000 products in 61 countries.

The manufacturers of homeopathic medications, like their counterparts in the allopathic pharmaceuticals industry, use sophisticated analytical techniques that ensure quality control and reproducibility. Their facilities are state of the art, including electronic controls and robotics whose automated functions can prepare the remedies more quickly than ever before. Purity of ingredients is of paramount importance. And packaging is designed for safety.

The Short of It: Long ago, they were hand-made by individual practitioners, but today they're standardized and made in high-tech labs under carefully monitored conditions—just like other pharmaceuticals.

Q. But they're not FDA regulated, are they?

The Long of It: Actually, the sale of homeopathic medicines has been regulated by the FDA (Food and Drug Administration) since the Federal Food, Drug and Cosmetic Act of 1938. Also, the marketing of homeopathic medicines is controlled by the FDA's *Compliance Policy Guide* of 1988, which provides labeling and sales guidelines. To qualify as a homeopathic medicine, according to the FDA, a remedy must be found in one of the official reference books that guide the preparation of homeopathic medicines, such as the widely used and accepted *HPUS (Homeopathic Pharmacopoeia of the United States)*. That's why you'll find the letters *HPUS* on a great deal of remedy packaging.

It is true that, despite all this, the FDA has not chosen to test homeopathic drugs for safety or efficacy. That's because the remedies are generally accepted as harmless. Many skeptics have called for testing, as has *Consumer Reports*. Homeopathy advocates would welcome this, but it seems the FDA has other priorities.

The Short of It: Yes, they are. But some people want to see more testing, and that would be great.

Q. Some of these substances are dangerous. How do you know you won't get poisoned?

The Long of It: Homeopathic medicines are so diluted that there is no chance of that occurring. In fact, if you really want to talk about dangerous drug use, let's look at some of the current problems that *are* FDA priorities.

Over 100,000 hospital patients die and over 2 million are injured every year by adverse reactions to prescription drugs (and that's *not* including cases where errors occur), and FDA officials are convinced the danger is growing.[5]

Another danger of conventional medicines is that with the growing number of formerly prescription drugs that are now available over-the-counter, many consumers are mixing drugs without being aware of possible adverse reactions to this "polypharmacy" approach.

The growing number of prescription drugs available over the Internet, with minimal physician "consultation," presents problems too.

The Short of It: You won't be harmed by the substances, since they are so diluted. You're more likely to experience problems with prescription drugs.

Q. Okay, if the remedies are so diluted, how can they be effective at all? Is it true there's sometimes "nothing" in them?

The Long of It: It's true that as yet no one understands the mechanism of how infinitesimal potencies of certain substances can heal. But we will know. Major strides are being made in research in this area—some by researchers interested in homeopathy, some by physicists, chemists, and molecular biologists who are pursuing related questions in their fields.

The idea that small amounts of substances can have a prolific impact is not exclusive to homeopathy. After all, human embryo development occurs as a result of extremely small amounts of genetic material. Mineral springs are another example, as they contain only tiny amounts of minerals. Even fluoride in drinking water is added in incredibly small dosages, with very evident results.

Of course, when we do learn the mechanism behind homeopathic doses, it will shake up the status quo. Radical new discoveries (such as those of Galileo, who challenged our vision of the cosmos, and Einstein, who challenged our notion of time) have a history of doing just this—so they may be unpopular for quite a while. But ultimately the curiosity so endemic to human nature wins out, and we come around.

The Short of It: Well, first you are worried the remedies are poisonous, and then you are worried they have nothing in them! Maybe you will try one for yourself one day and see what you think.

Q. Still, aren't you putting belief before science?

The Long *and* the Short of It: Seeing is believing. And observation is scientific. Homeopathy has two hundred years of solid empirical evidence on its side.

The Skeptical Spouse

The above questions and answers are meant to help Medicine Moms deal with curious or dubious friends, neighbors, and acquaintances. Yet perhaps one of the most common challenges faced by parents who are interested in changing the way they deal with their kids' health care is a co-parent reluctant to question conventional methods.

Although I have known it to be the other way around on occasion, it is generally moms who wish to convince dads to try something different (perhaps because many families consider children's health issues to fall primarily under mom's management, if not by convention than simply because sick kids tend to cry for "Mommy"). In fact, many Medicine Moms have told me that when they first broached the subject of homeopathy with their husbands, they more or less got asked if perhaps they'd been clobbered on the head with one too many of the kids' soccer balls.

Yet sooner or later, dads tend to come around. As the old Chinese aphorism says: "Man is the head of the family. Woman is the neck that turns the head."

Slowly and gently exposing your skeptical spouse to some of the information you've discovered can certainly help your cause. Relating "eyewitness" accounts of other satisfied parents' experiences with homeopathy can also be useful. But many Medicine Moms feel the most persuasive strategy of all is to ask a spouse to spend time (both the "quality" and the "quantity" kind) with the kids during their next few bouts with ear infection, bronchitis, or other common illness.

As one mom told me:

I don't think my husband really believed me about how hard our two-year-old daughter resisted taking the antibiotics she was often given for ear infections. He'd say, "Oh, come on. She's just a baby. Just pop a spoon in her mouth." I got pretty annoyed one day, and said, "Okay, this time it's your job." After a few fits (hers) and a few lapfuls of antibiotics (his), he asked me if there wasn't something else—anything!—we could try. Before that he'd thought I was crazy for wanting to give our daughter some little white homeopathic tablets. Now he said, "Hmm, she likes those!"

And as another recounted:

My child was bouncing of the wall from the inhalants he was taking for allergies and asthma. But my husband, who got home late during the week, often after the kids' bedtime, never got to see much of what I saw. I couldn't talk him into consulting a homeopath—until one weekend, which happened to be during peak allergy season, I had to go out of town. I came back to find my husband run ragged, not to mention feeling really badly for my son, who he said "hadn't seemed himself for days." The next week, my husband came with me to our new homeopathic doctor.

In both cases the rest of the story unfolded pretty much as you'd expect. Soon the spouses in question were Medicine Dads—and glad of it.

Be Careful What You Wish For

There is nothing wrong with healthy skepticism, nothing wrong with caution. As long as someone is even asking questions to begin with, it means they have an open mind. Maybe it's not wide open, but picture a back door opened just a crack. So, welcome questions—your own and other people's. In homeopathy, as in most other things, doubt is the beginning of faith.

One word of warning, however, when it comes to dealing with skeptics: Often total skeptics, once they've actually been exposed to homeopathy, become total fanatics. Soon your phone may be ringing off the hook with other kinds of questions—not doubting ones, but enthusiastic, inquisitive ones. "What do I do about this?" "Do you have any of that?"

If you find yourself in this position, the next chapter, devoted to some simple remedies—easy for "beginner" Medicine Moms to try out—is one you may want to share.

CHAPTER

5

Some Specifics

We are so fond of one another, because our ailments are the same.

—Jonathan Swift

lthough some people begin their involvement with home-opathy by consulting a professional right off the bat, many more seem to dip into it by tackling, on their own, a few simple symptoms—from a runny nose, to the bathroom "runs," to a minor rash or bruise. Such simple conditions are called *acute* and *self-limiting,* which means the body is likely to heal them on its own in good time. The reason people treat them is to promote healing sooner rather than later, and to bring relief for discomfort.

Homeopathy can give the body's healing powers a boost and speed the process along. But how does a novice know which home-opathic remedy to try for what ailment?

It's said that homeopathy treats people, not illnesses, and this is certainly the case. Nevertheless, over the course of many years of empirical research, it has been observed that certain specific remedies tend to work well with regards to particular symptoms in a majority of people. When you are starting with the modest ambition of relieving short-term symptoms, using these so-called "specifics" is as good a way to begin as any. Still, a potential Medicine Mom on this course may run into some confusing turns.

For one thing, if you were to go to a health food store or pharmacy and inspect the remedies there, you would notice that each bottle or tube listed one or two "indications," i.e., one or two uses for the remedy. But you may have heard of, or read of, a different use.

For example someone may have said you ought to try *sepia* for PMS irritability, but when you look at the *sepia* packaging, you see it is recommended for "stiff legs." Or you may have read *arsenicum* is useful for the beginning stages of a cold, but notice an indication for "diarrhea" on the package. In truth, one homeopathic remedy can have many uses and aid the body in coping with many symptoms. And if you were going to shop for your remedies in, say, France, you would not have these narrow guidelines to throw you off. Our FDA regulations, however, require that one or two primary indications be listed, and manufacturers comply. Alas, this can sometimes be more hindrance than help.

For another thing, you might run across a number of remedies all purporting to be useful in treating the same conditions, especially when it comes to things like "coughs" or "allergies." Indeed, numerous homeopathic remedies are useful for such common conditions—each in their own way. But neither all coughs nor all allergies are created equal. You might have a dry cough or a loose cough, a throat tickle in the morning, or an all-night bark. Similarly, an allergy may manifest itself primarily via watery eyes, or perhaps by postnasal drip, or perhaps by fatigue and facial puffiness. The trick is to know which remedy tends most often to match which symptom picture for most people.

Fortunately, we need not rely on remedy packaging, with its obvious limitations, to help us make our selections. Instead, there are two types of reference books that a Medicine Mom ought to know how to use and, ideally, have handy on her shelf.

Using a Repertory and a Materia Medica

The first type of book to get hold of is called a *repertory.* Repertories list detailed (very detailed!) symptoms in alphabetical order, and beside each symptom enumerate virtually every remedy recorded by homeopaths to have been effective in treating it. Some of the remedies will be listed in **BOLD CAPITAL LETTERS,** like so; and some will be listed in *lowercase italics,* like so. The remainder will be listed in regular type.

The **BOLD TYPE** indicates remedies that have been confirmed by the greatest number of practitioners; the *italics* indicate remedies that—while not confirmed in quite as many cases—are also frequently effective. Most beginners find these distinctions very helpful in deciding which remedy to try first. But try not to tune out the plain type remedies. The fact that they are listed means they have been known to work in some cases, and depending on the particular person needing treatment, they may well work in a given situation. To take your investigation to the next level, have a *materia medica* on hand. Once you have narrowed your search down to a remedy you'd like to try, or a few remedies among which you are deciding, you can look up each one (again, alphabetically) in this type of reference guide. The *materia medica* will provide a detailed picture of each remedy, explaining all the types of symptoms—both physical and emotional—it will impact. Reading about a remedy in this depth often confirms whether or not it is an appropriate choice.

Using two types of books may seem daunting at first, but Medicine Moms soon get the knack. In fact, I know many who enjoy thumbing through these books whenever they have a spare moment, and unearthing fascinating nuggets of information. Some, including myself, have even purchased computer CD-ROMs which combine both types of reference guides on one handy-dandy compact disk. (See the Resources section for recommendations on CD-ROMs, as well as on various editions of repertories and *materia medica*.)

Familiarizing yourself with reference guides is well worth the effort. However, as an introduction to some of the most common "household" remedies a Medicine Mom is most likely to encounter at the start of her homeopathic adventures, I have compiled a brief reference listing of my own. I call it *Mom's Mini Materia Medica*. It lists some common remedies and common usages for those remedies, and in many of the listings I've included an anecdote concerning either my firsthand experience with the remedy, or the experience of other Medicine Moms.

I hope all this will whet your appetite for more knowledge, but also trust that you will by no means take this listing as the final word in any health-related situation.

Before you read *Mom's Mini Materia Medica,* I also want to add the following cautions:

- Remember, homeopathy is helpful in the body's natural quest for balance. It enhances our own innate abilities to heal and to reach our potential for well-being. That potential, however, manifests itself differently in each of us. There is no more promise of a "cure" using homeopathy than there is with any other form of medicine.

- If you are self-treating, or treating a family member, for several months and the condition you are treating keeps recurring (even though it may recede temporarily), you ought to consult a professional homeopath. There could well be an underlying chronic imbalance that needs to be addressed with more long-term care. In general, one's overall health should improve when homeopathy is used. If that's not happening, explore further.

- Most important, never attempt to treat on your own any condition that is obviously serious or life-threatening in nature, e.g. profuse bleeding, obstructed breathing, chest pains, loss of consciousness, or injuries to the head, neck, or back. Moreover, as a parent you know when there is something very wrong with your child even if it does not appear on any list of serious symptoms. Never doubt your instincts in this area. If your child appears to be in trouble, get help immediately. Insist on it, even if others tell you it's not that big a deal.

Having said all that, I humbly offer my little guide to useful remedies for the common complaints of daily life. Please note: The remedies are listed by their full Latin names because this is the way their packaging is usually labeled.

Mom's Mini Materia Medica

Aconitum napellus: The Latin term for this monkshood plant comes from the root word meaning "dart." And that is just how *aconite* (as it is commonly referred to) works—quickly, deeply, and precisely. *Aconite* has many uses, including the treatment of fevers and colds, but the key thing I will always remember about *aconite* is that it rhymes with midnight. Like many kids, mine occasionally wakes in the *middle of the night* with a *high fever, seemingly from out of nowhere.* When this happens, especially if he is thirsty and agitated, I run for the cupboard and pull out this amazing remedy. If I get the jump on such symptoms, often by morning the upset all seems like a dream.

Agaricus muscarius: This fungus (known both as "crazy mushroom" and "Fly Agaric") is the prime homeopathic remedy for *frostbite,* and I know many "outdoors types" who keep it in their portable first aid kits. As with many homeopathic remedies, this one works most effectively when it is used early on. Break out your *agaricus* when you first feel numbness or cold spots in the extremities (feet and hands), or when you feel a prickly, needle-like sensation.

Allium cepa: I've said quite a bit about this one already. Made from red onion, it can work magic on a *runny nose with clear discharge that is typically caused by allergies.* It's made Medicine Moms out of many a skeptic. And it saves a fortune in tissues.

Alumina: A friend of mine was beside herself because her eleven-month-old had such bad *constipation* he hadn't had a bowel movement in five days. He was cranky as could be, pushing, straining, and crying. And she had exhausted all options, or so she thought. She called me and I leafed through my repertory, suggesting *alumina* (as the name suggests, it's from aluminum). Then my husband and I went out for the evening. When we got home there was an ecstatic message on our answering machine: "Billy pooped, Billy pooped!" (My husband just rolled his eyes. He is used to this sort of thing by now.)

Ambrosia artemis: This is ragweed, and another frequently touted *allergy* remedy. In my neck of the woods it works especially well in the autumn, whereas *Allium cepa* tends to be most effective in spring. But this may vary depending on what is in the air when, and of course on how an allergy manifests in a particular individual.

Antimonium tartaricum: There are many homeopathic remedies for coughs. You will get better at targeting the proper remedy after paying attention to the nuances of how a cough sounds and when it occurs.

For someone who has a great deal of *mucus in their chest but can't seem to bring it up,* and may *breathe with a gurgling sound* that can sometimes be heard across the room, this remedy (made from potassium salt of tartar emetic) may do the trick in terms of getting them to bring up what wouldn't come up before. Take it from me, it can work very rapidly. So if you give it to your kid, stand back—and wear something washable.

Apis mellifica: Made from the honeybee, it is the recommended remedy for *bee stings,* and I have seen it work wonders several times for one of my son's pals who is bee-prone. A few minutes after each episode, and a dose of *apis,* this child is back to his old self.

What's more, *apis* is effective for many kinds of *hives* and *skin eruptions.* If you know anyone who is *allergic to strawberries or shellfish,* but can't resist having a nibble now and then, they might want to have *apis* nearby.

Argentum nitricum: This is silver nitrate, a *diarrhea* remedy. However, you will want to use it for a particular kind of diarrhea—

the kind that accompanies the "nervous stomach" that comes from being very anxious about upcoming events—say getting up and speaking before a group of people, or waiting for some important news. Good to have on hand, especially if you or someone you love is the anxious type.

Another important note—this is the number one remedy for *baby colic.*

Arnica montana: At this point I barely know anyone who plays sports or works out who is not familiar with *arnica.* Usually they swear by it for *bruising* (i.e., any blunt trauma where the skin is not opened) and *overexertion of muscles. Arnica,* a mountain daisy, comes in creams and gels and is effective topically, but taken internally in homeopathic doses (not the herbal form!) it is even more miraculous. This remedy is excellent for those all too frequent occasions when your kids bash into something and you can see a red welt that you just know is going to evolve into a big black-and-blue mark. (In my household this generally happens the day before school pictures or visits from Grandma.) Soccer Moms, note: It's a favorite of the French national soccer team, for obvious reasons.

And moms, note for yourselves: *Arnica* is also great for *pain following childbirth* or *discomfort following overlifting* (like after giving the occasional piggy back ride).

Arsenicum album: Homeopathic medicines work best if you use them at the first sign of symptoms. *Arsenicum* is the remedy we try in my household at the *first sign of a cold.* Sometimes it can help our immune systems prevent it altogether, and sometimes it will lessen the impact.

This is also an astoundingly effective remedy for *traveler's diarrhea,* and my original homeopathic physician used to tell a story about endearing himself to a busload of fellow travelers in China by dispensing it after a particularly disruptive meal. Whenever my family takes a trip we literally don't leave home without it.

Perhaps you've noticed that the root of the word *arsenicum* is arsenic. That is indeed what this remedy is made from. But remember, this is an infinitesimal dose (indeed if you are using anything over 12C, there will not be any discernible remnant at all). Like cures like, and that is why a molecularly insignificant dose of a poison is just the thing for ridding the system of toxins.

Belladonna: As already mentioned, homeopathic doses of this "deadly nightshade" often convert the most skeptical parent when used to treat an *ear infection*. Not all ear infections respond to *belladonna,* but many do when the symptom picture includes *fever with rapid onset* and *flushed cheeks.*

In my household *belladonna* has, more than once, saved the day.

Bryonia: Made from wild hops, *bryonia* is perhaps best known for treating *headaches*. But it is also a common remedy for a *dry cough.* I find it very handy because I can give it to my son for his cough and take it myself for the headache I got from listening to the cough.

Calendula: From the garden marigold, this remedy, like *arnica,* has become exceedingly well known. Many households have it handy in gel or ointment form, but taken in homeopathic pellets it is even more effective for promoting healing of *cuts and abrasions.* In my experience, it can really bring comfort to kids with *skin chapped from the cold* or *noses raw from blowing.*

I live near the beach and can also attest *calendula* has given many friends and neighbors relief from wicked *sunburns.*

Cantharsis: It's made from Spanish fly, but don't get any funny ideas. It's yet another great *burn* or *sunburn* remedy, especially if you are starting to *blister. Cantharsis* is also a common remedy for *bladder infections.*

Carbo vegetalis: This is charcoal, and it's for *digestive disturbances* such as bloating, belching, and—excuse me—passing *foul-smelling gas.* Let's face it, we could all use it sometime.

Causticum: This is potassium hydrate and is used in conditions affecting the central nervous system. For everyday purposes, it is a great remedy for *stiff neck* (an affliction I myself often suffer from as I hunch over my computer keyboard). It is also used to treat *carpal tunnel syndrome,* but this is one of those conditions I would certainly want to consult a professional on.

Chamomilla: This is the chamomile flower, used medicinally by so very many cultures around the world for centuries. You already know that, in homeopathic doses, it is a fantastic *teething* remedy. It can help with *earache* as well (and indeed sometimes earaches are related to teething).

Chamomilla is also good for *restlessness,* and *irritability* in general, and is a common remedy for *colic.* When a baby is too fussy and fretful to sleep, and instead wants you to carry him around all night, supplement your TLC with a little *chamomilla*—and then try a dose yourself. Sweet dreams!

China officinalis: This is cinchona, or Peruvian bark. If you have any condition that is accompanied by a *great loss of fluids* (diarrhea, continuous vomiting, even sweating a great deal), this remedy will quickly restore body balance. (Obviously you should also rehydrate as quickly as possible.)

Cocculus indicus: From the fruit of the Indian cockle tree, this works well for *motion sickness* in cars and airplanes. We never take our son on a flight without it, and if the stewardesses knew what we were sparing them, they'd thank us. An extra benefit: It's also the prime homeopathic remedy for *jet lag,* so for the air traveler this is "one-stop shopping."

Coffea cruda: If you are sleepless in Seattle—or anywhere else—try this remedy, which I am sure you have already guessed is made from coffee beans (although they are unroasted). It will be especially helpful if the *sleeplessness* occurs from the result of being "wound up" or "jazzed" with excitement. I recently took it when I was happy and excited about a workshop I would be teaching the next day—knowing if I didn't get some rest I would burn out before the event had actually begun.

Coffea is also a remedy used for relief of *toothache.*

Cuprum metallicum: When a neighbor's very athletic son kept complaining of *charley horses,* nothing seemed to help, except this remedy—which is copper. It worked like a charm. In general, it's useful for any *spasmodic pain.*

Drosera rotundifolia: This is the sundew plant. It is another frequently recommended *cough* remedy. Remember, you may well have to try a few to hit the right one for a particular cough. But this one seems to work best on those annoying ticklings which turn into hackings starting in the *middle of the night.* I keep it in my bedside table along with my *aconite.*

Equisetum hiemale: A gentle and effective remedy for occasional *bed-wetting.* What can a Medicine Mom say but, "Hooray!"

Euphrasia: Commonly known as "eyebright" (which just about sums it up), this remedy is for *eye irritation,* be it from allergy, pollutants, or contact lens wear. You can take it internally, like all the other remedies.

I also highly recommend an eye drop called Optique®, by Boiron, which contains *euphrasia* and a few other goodies and comes in one-dose dispensers. I have worn contacts for decades, and tried every eye drop known to man. Each only made my eyes *more* irritated—until I found this.

Ferrum phosphoricum: You know how sometimes your kids will come down with low-grade fevers but yet nothing else seems wrong with them? It's always sort of baffling, and one never knows quite what to do. Maybe they are in the first stage of a cold or some other sort of viral infection, which may or may not bloom. This remedy (iron phosphate) is the one to try, as it is for *fevers of unknown origin.* With its help, sometimes what may have bloomed simply fades away. In such cases, the gentle homeopathic intervention has prevented the body from having to generate more extreme symptoms to correct its slight imbalance.

Gelsemium sempervirens: This California jasmine is aesthetically lovely, a climbing flower with long leaves and yellow petals. When used as a homeopathic remedy, it is even lovelier. It can really help *shorten and mitigate the course of the flu,* and last winter got my son back to school before most of his classmates when the bug hit.

(Also very effective for the flu, is Oscillococcinum®. "Oscillo," as it's known, is the best-selling over-the-counter *flu* medicine in France and is rapidly catching on here via word of mouth. If taken at the first sign of chills, aches, etc., I have seen it stop a flu in its tracks.)

Hepar sulphuris: This remedy is a type of calcium sulphide. Although often used in homeopathy to stimulate the *ripening of abscesses or boils,* it is also good for yeast *discharge,* and for *sore throats that are primarily in the left side of the throat.*

Hydrastis canadensis: This is goldenseal, and it is one remedy that really showed me the difference between herbal and homeopathic treatments. Years ago, unable to clear up a wicked sinus infection with conventional antibiotics, I tried a recommended tea made from goldenseal root. It cleared me up within twenty-four hours, enabling me to breathe normally for the first time in six weeks. There were side effects, however. The herb caused intestinal upset, and left me fatigued. Nevertheless, I used it on occasion when similar symptoms occurred. Then about two years ago I had badly *blocked sinuses* again. This time the tea proved ineffective. I called my homeopath and he suggested homeopathic *hydrastis,* which is the same substance in a diluted, infinitesimal dose. Not

only did it work instantly, it spared me any unpleasant consequences.

Hypericum perforatum: Ever inadvertently slam a door or
drawer on your fingers—or someone else's? I have! Before the resulting screams get the neighbors dialing 911, give *hypericum* (St.
John's wort), which is a wonderful acute *painkiller.* Indeed, it is also
good as an emergency intervention for any *sharp, shooting pain*
(from one caused by a slipped disk to one caused by an animal
bite). Naturally, you will want to have a thorough exam of the affected area as soon as possible, but *hypericum* makes the trip to—
and the wait at—the emergency room far more bearable.

Ignatia amara: This remedy is St. Ignatius' bean, the seed of a
climbing shrub called *strychnos ignati.* (And yes, that plant contains strychnine, but as with the *arsenicum* remedy there is only an
infinitesimal amount in any remedy under 12C, and no molecular
trace above that potency.)

Ignatia is one of those remedies one hopes one will never have
to use. That is because it is good for mitigating a *state of shock* that
comes from getting a big fright, or from learning grief-inducing
news. Nevertheless, it cannot hurt to keep some on hand. I have
even used it on my son when he has awoken from an upsetting
nightmare with his heart racing and had trouble calming down.

Ipecac: Here's a remedy recommended for *nausea,* and also
one with which it is easy to demonstrate the principles of homeopathy at work. We've all heard of Ipecac syrup to induce vomiting (for
example, after swallowing a toxin). Since this substance (from a
Brazilian shrub) in a large dose causes vomiting in a well person, it
would—according to the Law of Similars—*relieve vomiting* and
nausea in an unwell person if taken in a tiny homeopathic dose.
Granted, sometimes throwing up is just what we need to do. But
homeopathic *ipecac* is useful in situations where profuse vomiting

threatens to cause dehydration, or when *vomiting is not relieving feelings of nausea* (as in *morning sickness*).

Kali bichronicum: Our family homeopath says, "If it sticks, use *Kali bich.*" Now this is one of our standard household mantras. Made from potassium bichromae, this remedy is for when the *mucus* that's coming out of a nose is *thick* and *yellow-green,* and makes your kids (and you) want to say "Yuck." (When the mucus becomes clear again, we go back to *arsenicum album.*)

Kali muriaticum: This is potassium chloride and was recommended to us by our homeopath when there was *fluid behind the ear but no infection.*

Kali phosphoricum: This is potassium bichromate, and at my house we call it "the homework remedy." That is because it is good for relieving symptoms associated with *mental exhaustion* from extended intellectual work or study (such symptoms include *headache* and *short-term memory depletion*—as, for example, when you cram so hard for a test you temporarily can't seem to recall a thing). In today's typical household, it seems like parents are often as stressed out by homework than kids are (if not more so). So keep a dose handy for yourself when those incomprehensible math problems or "make-a-shoebox-diorama" instructions come home in your child's backpack.

Lachesis: This remedy (made from the venom of the South American Bushmaster snake—and yes, very, very diluted) is a good *sore throat* remedy *especially if the pain seems to alternate sides of the throat and/or the pains from the throat seem to spread into the ear.* As with coughs, sore throats come in many shapes and sizes. You may need to try a few remedies before finding the one that is right for the particular sore throat symptoms of an individual at a particular time. (Of course, unlike with coughs, moms can't hear the evidence for themselves. With small children, see if you can get them to point to where it hurts. Older ones can describe it better in words, especially once you get them used to being specific about their symptoms.)

Ledum palustre: This is wild rosemary and I've seen it work wonders on *insect bites*. Once, a friend's son's leg was so badly swollen from a bug bite, she made a pediatrician's appointment. Then she gave her son *ledum* on the way to the doctor's. By the time they got to the office, the swelling was gone, the bite invisible—and the pediatrician thought my friend was a raging hypochondriac.

Lycopodium clavatum: This is another one of those don't-leave-home-without-it remedies. Made from the spores of the club moss plant, it can work wonders for *traveler's constipation* (and I'll spare you my anecdote).

Lycopodium actually has many additional uses. It, too, is a *sore throat* remedy (when the pain starts out on the right and then switches to the left). And it is good for most *complaints that tend to worsen between 4 P.M. and 8 P.M.* (take note if you have a *baby that's especially fussy* at this time).

Magnesia phosphorica: Medicine Moms, this one is for you. Made from magnesium phosphate, many women find it a wonderful treatment for relief of *menstrual cramps*. Indeed, I have some friends who have tried all kinds of herbal concoctions for cramps, to no avail, but have had considerable success with this gentle homeopathic remedy.

Mercurius dulcis: This is calomel and it's recommended for *swimmer's ear*. It's a summertime staple at our house.

Mercurius vivus or Mercurius solubilis: These are both forms of mercury (the first metallic mercury, the second a mixture of mercury ammonium devised by Hahnemann). They are said to work the same and are recommended for some *sore throat* (when the whole throat is sore, as opposed to one side) and for *canker sores* that are *inside the mouth.*

Natrum muriaticum: The is sea salt. It's recommended for *canker sores outside the mouth* (the kind when you're sure the whole world is staring). For me, this remedy was also successful in alleviating *dry eye* syndrome which, as anyone who has ever had it knows, can be excruciating. (By now, you can no doubt see how this remedy illustrates homeopathic principles. While ingesting a large quantity of salt would cause water retention, a homeopathic dose will help the eyes to tear.)

Nux vomica: Made from poison chestnut (again, don't worry, it's nontoxic in highly diluted homeopathic form), this is an excellent remedy for *indigestion* (bloating, gas, *constipation*) after overeating rich, fatty foods. I keep it handy around the holidays. Oh, who am I kidding? I always keep it handy.

Phosphorus: This is another *cough* remedy. On my son it works well when I can really hear the cough is from *deep in the chest*). It is often doctor recommended for *lung conditions.*

Podophyllum peltatum: Made from the roots of the mayapple plant, this is another *diarrhea* remedy—and one that tends to work very well on kids and on teething infants. There are a number of diarrhea remedies, but this is often the one to use when you hear that loud rumbling sound just before the big event.

Pulsitilla: This is the wind flower, and another oft-used remedy for *allergy symptoms* (I find it works well when one's nose alternates between stuffiness and runniness) and *sinusitis*. Sometimes it, too, is recommended to treat *ear infections,* especially those *not accompanied by high fever.*

Rhus toxicodendron: This is poison ivy, and recommended for treating *itchy skin rashes.* My husband is so susceptible to poison ivy that exposure to it in its natural state has actually landed him in the hospital, so our homeopath has recommended that he take a homeopathic dose of *Rhus tox,* anytime he thinks he might be in danger of exposure to the plant itself. So far—fingers crossed—this has been very helpful. He has still contracted rashes a couple of times, but with the homeopathic preventative, they have been much less severe.

Ruta graveolens: This remedy (from the rue or bitterwort plant) is good for injuries to the soft tissue that go a bit deeper than the surface bruises that call for *arnica.* It is good, for example, for *tennis elbow* and for *injuries of the knee and Achilles tendon.* My husband once had to spend a day showing out-of-town relatives around New York City while nursing an Achilles injury. Were it not for *ruta,* he would have given out halfway through Central Park.

Another good use of *ruta* is for eye strain, so computer jockeys should always have some on hand.

Sepia: This is ink of the cuttlefish or giant squid. It's often recommended for *postpartum* blues and blahs, and I use it, with good results, for *PMS*—as do many of my friends. It may sound odd to you—it sure did to me—that this substance could have such a salutary effect on mood. Years ago squid ink was used as a pigment in paints. Artists would moisten the tips of their brushes with saliva, ingesting some of the ink in the process, and then develop fatigue, irritability, and depression. Of course, as homeopathic principles have it, taken in an infinitesimal dose, *sepia* has the opposite effect.

Silicea: I don't know about your kids, but when mine gets a splinter, he is not exactly a stoic about it. Trying to remove one can bring on a fit of epic proportions. If it doesn't look infected, we often just give him some *silicea,* which has a remarkable ability to help the body push the *splinter* out on its own. *Silicea* is made from pure flint prepared from quartz crystal.

Spongia tosta: This is toasted sea sponge, good for the kind of *coughs* that are *hacking, barking, and croupy.* It's a good one to try if the cough is *exhausting, going on day and night.* It took me a while to discover *spongia,* but now I can instantly recognize the exact sound my son makes when he needs it. Again, treating coughs takes practice and patience. You may well want professional help as you find your way.

Staphysagria: This is the Stavesacre, or larkspur plant. It is an excellent remedy for *mosquito bites,* and can also be used preventatively. You can take a dose daily when in known mosquito terrain. Alas, I found out about this one too late. Last summer my son scratched his mosquito bites so hard he came down with a nasty case of impetigo. You wouldn't want that to happen to anyone in your family, believe me.

Another use for *staphysagria* is to help deal with head lice, which as you may be aware is increasingly becoming a problem. Along with all the usual hygienic measures for a case of head lice, a homeopath may recommend *staphysagria* in a very low potency. However, this is one of those situations in which a professional should be consulted, both to make sure you have the correct potency and because there are other remedies that may be given before or after *staphysagria* to help correct a particular individual's propensity for getting head lice in the first place.

Sulphur: *Sulphur* is, obviously enough, from the mineral of the same name. It is often the right remedy for *rashes, eczema,* and *other skin conditions where there is itching and burning.*

Symphytum officinale: Often skeptics have asked me, "Well, you wouldn't treat a broken bone with homeopathy, would you?"

Well, no. That is, not exclusively. Obviously a broken bone needs to be set, and the venue for doing that is usually an emergency room or a conventional doctor's office. But when the fracture is healing, an excellent way to speed the process is to give this remedy, which is made from comfrey.

Tabacum: The first time my family and I went on a cruise ship, I was told one virtually never felt *seasickness* on these things. Hah! Two days later some choppy seas had half the ship on Dramamine. But not us. We took this very effective remedy, which is tobacco in homeopathic potency.

Veratrum album: This is another *diarrhea* remedy. I use it as my backup to *Arsenicum album.* The latter tends to work better if the cause is food poisoning, but if I have a twenty-four-hour stomach virus, then *Veratrum album* (which is white hellebore) tends to do the trick. Of course it's hard to determine the immediate cause when one is first in the grips of this condition, so I like to have both remedies handy.

Zincum metallicum: *Zinc* is recommended for hangovers, especially from drinking too much wine. It's also good even if you've had just a little wine, but are sensitive to it. I think I'll coyly decline to tell you any firsthand anecdotes regarding this remedy.

Hitting the Bull's-Eye

In homeopathy there is a term called "finding the *simillimum.*" This refers to zeroing in on the remedy that precisely matches the symptom picture you are attempting to treat. When it does happen—and sometimes it does simply due to a fortuitous combination of beginner's luck and solid instincts—the results can be breathtakingly swift. Poof! Symptoms seem to subside as if by divine intervention. But hitting the bull's-eye in this way is not always possible, and indeed certainly not always necessary. So please don't spend too much time obsessing on whether you've got every detail covered in terms of which substance corresponds to which symptoms, or on whether to try this remedy or that one first.

If something isn't working within twenty-four hours, you can simply try your second choice. But often this won't be required. Happily, most of us will respond well to a range of remedies. Like cures like, but a remedy needn't be exactly tuned to each and every nuance of an illness to instigate healing. There is a spectrum of similarity among similars, and if you are even in the ballpark, you may well see a positive result.

About Combination Remedies

Another thing you may be wondering about is whether or not to use combination remedies, which of late have become so prominently marketed. Among professional homeopaths there has been, and continues to be, much debate about this topic—with many "classical" homeopaths resisting the trend and protesting that combinations have not been proven in the Hahnemannian way. The arguments sometimes veer, as they do in many professions, from the practical to the philosophical and the political. And each side may accuse the other of not being "true" to the calling.

As in the case of chaos theory and quantum physics, this is all very interesting intellectually, but on a nuts-and-bolts level not so compelling. Being a common sense advocate above all, I like to do what works, and what is simplest. And most Medicine Moms I know agree that combinations can certainly work in *some* instances, and may save a good deal of time otherwise spent hunting around.

In *Mom's Mini Materia Medica* I have already mentioned Optique® eye drops, which is a combination of numerous remedies that have a beneficial effect on the eyes, including *euphrasia, calendula* and *Kali muriaticum*. Another combination I have used with success is Hyland's Diarrex®, a diarrhea remedy that combines *arsenicum* with *phosphorus, Mercurius vivus,* and other ingredients. As the mother of an active boy, I am also fond of Boiron's Arnicalm® Trauma, which combines *arnica* with *ledum* and *Bellis perennis* (English daisy). The latter two ingredients are good for deep healing of black eyes, bruises and sprains, and are often recommended to follow an initial course of *arnica.* Having them all in one remedy appeals to my never-ending quest for efficiency.

There are also numerous homeopathic combination formulas which are marketed for relief of symptoms of allergies, common colds, sinusitis, and even stress and fatigue. Will they work for you and your family? Perhaps. But the only way to know for sure is to try. Homeopathic combinations are formulated to treat the most commonly occurring symptoms of these conditions as they manifest in the greatest number of people. So, long story short, they work for some people some of the time. If they don't work for you in any given situation, that does not mean homeopathy won't work—only that you should try something more specific.

In addition to exploring combination remedies, you may want to take a look at some of the remedy kits that are for sale. They offer various selections of specific remedies—with some of the smaller ones being tailored to themes such as children's kits, sports kits, travel kits, and first aid kits. These kits make it easy to store, find, and transport remedies, and mean fewer late-night trips to the pharmacy. In my estimation, they are well worth the initial investment.

How Much, How Often, and How?

Now we get to the question of what dosage to take, how often remedies should be taken, and in what manner they should be taken. Sometimes practitioners vary in their advice on this subject, and if you are seeing one, you should certainly abide by his recommendations, as he will be most familiar with your circumstances and can individualize treatment. What I am going to tell you, however, is generally customary, and is the way I was instructed by my original practitioner.

When you look at the labeling of each and every homeopathic remedy, you will find its Latin name followed by a number and letter, most commonly 6C, 12C, or 30C. These letters and numbers indicate how many times a remedy has been diluted and succussed (which, you'll recall, means vigorously shaken). The higher the number, the more dilutions and succussions—and the stronger the remedy. For the most part, it's recommended that acute symptoms be treated with 30C and chronic complaints with 6C or 12C. Since acute complaints are what you will likely be treating (remember, chronic ones ought best be treated by a professional), you can purchase remedies accordingly.

You should be aware that remedies also come in even higher dilutions, such as 200C. These are usually not on display, but kept "behind the counter" at pharmacies. Though they are not prescription, they must be requested. There is good reason for making them less available, for they should be used with caution. With a 200C you really need to know what you are doing, and be as certain as you can that the symptom picture and the remedy match up. Also, if used on a highly sensitive person, or given too frequently, a 200C strength remedy, even if it is the bull's-eye remedy, might cause an "aggravation"—which means the symptoms get accentuated before they recede. This can certainly be unnerving for a beginner, and reason enough to stick with 30C for the time being.

As for how often a 30C remedy should be taken, usually three to four times a day is sufficient. You can strengthen the effect of any remedy by giving it more often. But again, I wouldn't do this without a practitioner's input at first.

When it comes to actually taking the remedies, most packaging recommends you take three to five pellets dry and let them melt in your mouth. Another way of doing it is to put a pellet in four ounces of water, let it melt, and take a tablespoon of that mixture three or four times a day. (You need fewer pellets in water, because—according to homeopathic principles—dilution makes a remedy stronger.) The mixture itself can be used for twenty-four hours, so you can take all your day's dosages from the one mix.

Many Medicine Moms like to give their kids remedies in this manner as it's often easier to get a little one to sip a bit of water than to suck on pellets. (This is how my son and his pals came up with the "magic water" phrase mentioned earlier.) The water method initially presented a bit of a problem for me in that it did not seem as portable as the dry pellet method. But then I learned this Medicine Mom trick: Take a couple of pellets and dilute them in a water bottle with a sipper top (approximately one pellet for each four ounces of water). Carry that with you, and give a sip as a dose. For good measure, you can give the bottom of the bottle a few whacks with the palm of your hand (i.e., a few extra succussions) before each dose.

One important note, however: When taking a remedy as a preventative—e.g., *Rhus tox* before poison ivy exposure, or *staphysagria* before exposure to mosquitos—do not take it in water. Always take a preventative dry, allowing a few pellets to melt on the tongue.

What Interferes with Remedies?

Another area in which there are some differences of opinion in the field of homeopathy is what substances, if any, may prevent remedies from being their most effective. Among the substances patients are often warned off while using homeopathy are coffee, mint (including mint toothpastes and teas), chocolate, and spicy foods (including garlic and onion).

Considering the minute dosages of homeopathic remedies, one can see why it has been suspected by Hahnemann and followers that strong tastes and/or stimulants might overpower their impact. Nevertheless, there is no clinical proof I'm aware of that such substances have a detrimental effect on homeopathic healing.

My own practitioner took a commonsense approach to this issue, which I now pass along to you.

- In general, here is a simple guideline: It's best not to eat or drink anything fifteen minutes before or after taking a remedy—and if there is an especially strong taste in your mouth, wait until it is gone.
- As for coffee, it obviously won't be a problem for your kids, but if you like a cup of coffee in the morning and want to take a remedy yourself, wait at least an hour. (By the way, if you'd like to quit coffee with some homeopathic help, remember *chamomilla,* or try *coffea,* which as you already know is made from the coffee bean itself.)
- As for mint, it's likely this prohibition began because in Hahnemann's day people used an excessive amount of mint to mask the foul odors that resulted from sub-par hygiene. Many practitioners believe it's not a problem in modest amounts, so don't throw out your Tic Tacs®. Just don't use a mint breath freshener or toothpaste right before or after taking a remedy. If this is a problem for you, there are homeopathic toothpastes that omit mint altogether.

In addition to avoiding certain substances, I have heard it said that one should never carry homeopathic remedies through an airport metal detector. From personal experience (I schlep them everywhere), and the experience of fellow Medicine Moms (who hate to be far from home without their remedies), I can attest to the overzealousness of this advice. My remedies are as helpful when I get to my destination as they were when I left home, metal detectors notwithstanding.

Another thing one often hears is not to touch the medicated pellets with one's fingertips, nor place them on any surface. This warning originated when all of the medicinal substance was on the outside of the pellet and could easily be rubbed off. Nowadays sophisticated manufacturing techniques (Boiron, for example, has a patented triple impregnation method) lead to a more even distribution of remedy throughout the pellet. But common sense still must prevail, and needless to say you don't want to handle these any more than you have to. Fortunately there's little need to overhandle the medicines, since another recent manufacturing advance has led to dispensers that shake individual pellets loose with relative ease. However, if you do brush one with your index finger, or drop it on your shirt, don't be overly concerned.

There is such a thing as being *too* careful—and that's generally not good for one's health.

CHAPTER

6

What's the Difference? Homeopathy (versus Allopathy) for Common Conditions

The desire to take medicine is perhaps the greatest feature which distinguishes man from animals.
—Sir William Osler, Canadian physician

Now that you possess quite a few useful nuggets of knowledge about certain common homeopathic remedies and how to take them, this is a good moment to expand on the reasons Medicine Moms often give homeopathic remedies in lieu of (or occasionally alongside) conventional prescription or popular over-the-counter remedies. In this chapter, I am going to go over some very common ailments and discuss the differences in the two approaches.

I certainly do not mean to indicate that the homeopathic way is always the right way, to the exclusion of any other ways. But the homeopathic and allopathic approaches generally come at the same things from divergent perspectives, and it's always nice to be able to justify—to yourself and, yes, to those skeptics—what you are doing and why.

Remember, skeptics have a right to their questions, opinions, and doubts. But a doubting mother-in-law or next-door neighbor is less likely to make you second-guess yourself if you really have facts at your fingertips. With that in mind, let's discuss some of the most common medical conditions that are likely to affect your children at one time or another, and compare the homeopathic approach with the more standard approach.

The Dreaded Fever—But Should It Be Dreaded?

I remember the first time my son was running a fever. I put my hand to his forehead and felt the warmth, then rushed to confirm what I already knew with one of those in-your-ear thermometers.

Even though I'd heard those weren't always accurate, I treated its pronouncement of 102.6° as if it were the word from heaven on high, and I just about knocked my husband over rushing for the Tylenol®. In the next few hours I probably poked my poor child in the ear with that thermometer at least a dozen times. I monitored each fraction of a degree of his temperature, all the while clucking like an adrenaline-crazed mother hen.

Over the next year or so, whenever I'd call my pediatrician and say "my son has a fever," he would reinforce my behavior by instructing me to give him "a good dose" of acetaminophen. Then one day my son got a fever while my pediatrician was away. A backup doctor returned one of my fevered "fever calls" and took a somewhat different tact.

"Well, is your son uncomfortable?" he asked.

"Why, no," I replied. "As a matter of fact he is dancing along with Barney at the moment."

"Is he having difficulty breathing?"

"Uh, no . . . he's singing."

"Anything else the matter other than fever?"

"Uh . . . nope."

"Hmm, well, you say your thermometer says . . ."

"One hundred and one, point nine!"

"Well, you know, you can give him something if it makes *you* feel better, but fever is the body's way of fighting something off. You may want to just keep an eye on it for a while and see if anything develops."

This world-rocking piece of advice really gave me pause. But in truth, I think I gave my son more Tylenol® anyway—just to make *myself* feel better.

Later, however, my explorations of homeopathy compelled me to revisit this issue. A little reading on the topic reminded me that the body responds to infection with fever because increased body temperature heightens the body's natural defense mechanisms, enabling it to manufacture additional specialized white blood cells (called leucocytes). These cells destroy bacteria and viruses, and remove irritants and damaged tissue from the body. Squelch the fever, inhibit the healing response.

As I've mentioned, homeopathy does indeed have many remedies for fever. Among them are:

Aconite (for fever of sudden onset)
Belladonna (when the face is very flushed)
Ferrum phos (for mild fevers of unknown origin)

So, you may be wondering: Isn't homeopathy dealing with fever the same way as allopathy—that is, by trying to make it go away? The answer is no. In homeopathy, the goal of a fever remedy is not to stifle the fever but to resolve the underlying condition that is leading to the fever. With the right remedy, the fever can "break" naturally—and sometimes does very quickly—because the totality of the underlying issue has been addressed.

Besides, as a parent, I know it is difficult to "do nothing" when your child has a fever—even if you have the sort of pediatrician who quite reasonably advises a wait-and-see approach in situations where the fever is not too high and the child is not uncomfortable. Giving a child with a fever a homeopathic remedy allows a parent to "do something," and it is something that can make both parent and child feel better in the short as well as the long run.

The Uncommon Cold (and Cough)

I know, I know—that snuffly, runny, sneezy, wheezy condition we all know so well is generally referred to as the "common" cold. Yet my family and I have had many a cold and I can tell you—as I'm sure you can tell me—how different one is from another.

Some colds make you feel as if your head is stuffed full of cotton; some make you feel like there's a faucet in your nose. Some center right in the middle of your chest; some seem to affect one side of your face and head but not the other. Some colds are practically incapacitating; some merely mildly annoying. Some colds come with postnasal drips, sore throats, and coughs; others have fewer embellishments. Some colds seem to linger, while others are more quickly dispatched.

What is "common" about these colds, and what do these colds have "in common"? Not much. Yet when we make the ritualistic trip to the drugstore cold medicine aisle, we are met with an arsenal of over-the-counter cold "relievers" that are not in any way specifically geared for our particular cold *du jour.*

Moreover, we are faced with many products whose sole function—catchy names and marketing claims aside—is to suppress all of our irritating symptoms. What's wrong with that, you may ask?

Remember, every symptom is part of the body's attempt to heal itself. The purpose of a sneeze, a cough, or a runny nose is to expel toxins from the body. If we take decongestants and antihistamines, cough suppressants and whatnot, we've plugged up nearly every outlet the body has for healing itself. Throw a prescription antibiotic in there (as far too many of us are wont to do in the face of a severe cold) and the counterproductive job we've done is complete. Now the cold will take far longer to resolve itself than it would have if we had simply left the body alone.

But in the face of colds, as with fevers, we want to do something. And fortunately, homeopathy does give us some things to do. Among the remedies already mentioned with regards to colds are:

Arsenicum album (good for runny noses with clear discharge and, if taken early enough, sometimes able to head off a cold at the onset)

Hydrastis (for sinuses so plugged that breathing through the nose seems nearly impossible)

Kali bich (for colds with thick, sticky mucus)

I also have seen good results from Coldeeze®, a widely marketed cold lozenge using zinc in a homeopathic potency, which diminishes the length and severity of lingering colds.

Among those mentioned with regards to coughs are:

Antimonium tart (when one cannot seem to bring up mucus in the lungs)
Bryonia (for a dry cough)
Drosera (for the middle-of-the-night coughs that start as tickles and turn into hacks)
Phosphorus (for coughs that come from deep in the chest and sound "gurgly")

You will find many additional symptom-tailored remedies listed in any repertory.

Finding the remedy that most closely matches the precise symptoms that a cold manifests in a particular person will—as the over-the-counter remedies do—offer some relief. But with homeopathy, the relief that is offered comes from the fact that the body's own defenses are being activated against the virus that is most likely causing the cold in the first place. (And in the case of a cough, a remedy may resolve it by having the body expel the mucus that is causing the cough. This is very helpful indeed—though one should be prepared to run a load of wash.)

Does this mean a Medicine Mom needs to swear off allopathic over-the-counter cold medicines forever? To be honest, I have done this for the most part—but not altogether.

I might use an over-the-counter suppressant medication once in a while—and very sparingly—in a special circumstance to temporarily relieve a symptom that is truly getting in the way of some vital function. For example, if my son can hardly breathe and can't sleep because of it, I may supplement his homeopathic course of treatment with one dose of a nighttime cold liquid before bed. If I need to do some public speaking and don't want to have to blow my nose for a few hours, I may take an over-the-counter decongestant that will last me for that brief duration.

But I know from having learned the hard way that if I overdo such methods, they will not only cease giving me any relief, but will cause a "backlash" effect that worsens the symptoms and drags out the whole miserable cold experience.

Have you ever, for example, taken a lot of nasal spray during a cold to open up your nasal passages? It feels wonderful at first—blessed deliverance! But then you need to do it more and more frequently, until you find yourself doing it far more often than the directions recommend. The next thing you know, you feel like a nasal spray junkie. And worst of all, the product has ceased to do for you what it started out doing.

That was one "quick fix" that ends up getting you in a fix. But this sort of thing is simply not going to happen if you use primarily homeopathic remedies to treat your "uncommon colds."

Sore Throats

When it comes to sore throats, generally the most we can expect from that aforementioned drugstore aisle is a little relief in the form of a soothing lozenge. Those certainly can't do anyone much harm, but using a homeopathic remedy as well can get to the root of the problem and help the body correct the imbalance that is creating the throat pain.

Like cold and cough remedies, these tend to be quite symptom-specific, since sore throats can really vary as to how they are sore and where they are sore. Some sore throat remedies listed in *Mom's Mini Materia Medica* are:

Hepar sulph (for when the soreness is primarily left-sided)

Lachesis (for when the pain seems to alternate sides of the throat and/or shoot into the ears)

Lycopodium (for when the pain starts out on the right, but then relocates to the left and stays there)

Mercurius sol or *viv* (for when the whole throat is sore)

And of course, any repertory will list some others as well.

One caveat: If you have been using throat lozenges, wait fifteen minutes or so after sucking on the lozenge before taking the homeopathic remedy so as not to have a lingering strong flavor on the mouth.

Earaches

A lot has already been said about ear troubles in this book, but to briefly recap: Not every earache means there is an ear infection; not every ear infection is bacterial; and even ear infections that are bacterial need not always call for antibiotics (which can, in the long run, do more harm than good).

The foregoing facts are well established, and widely reported even in the most mainstream medical publications. Unfortunately, the tendency of many pediatricians is to take the "road most traveled," prescribing antibiotics even if there is nothing more than a bit of redness in—or a bit of fluid behind—the ear.

Studies have shown that gentle homeopathic ear remedies are often extremely effective. And needless to say, they do not present the dire risk that overexposure to antibiotics can.

Are all earaches created equal? Of course not. They have differing causes, and differing symptoms. Some specific remedies include:

Belladonna (when accompanied by fever with flushed face)
Chamomilla (when ear pain in a child is accompanied by much irritability and the child wants to be carried all the time; when earache is related to teething)
Kali mur (when there is some fluid behind the ear but no infection)
Mercurius dulcis (for swimmer's ear)
Pulsitilla (when the ear feels painful or stuffy, but there is no fever and the face has a pallor rather than a flush)

It's perfectly understandable if parents want to consult with a doctor when a young child has an earache, even if they are not fans of antibiotics. You may want the doctor to check to see if there is an object in the ear, just to be on the safe side (a rare event, but not unheard of for little ones with an experimental bent).

What the doctor will do, as you most likely know, is use an otoscope—a simple viewing instrument with a magnifying lens and a light to examine the ear's interior. This is an excellent point at which to ask exactly what he sees (and maybe convince him to let you have a peek, as my current pediatrician will gladly do). Now the relative severity of the situation can be assessed and you can make your decision accordingly. Remember, it is, in fact, your decision in the end, and as you learn more, you will gain the confidence to make such decisions, and make them well.

P.S. You can purchase an otoscope for yourself, if you are so inclined. They are available through many "kid stuff" mail order catalogs that are probably even now stuffing your mailbox.

Allergies

As with over-the-counter cold medications, many over-the-counter and prescription allergy medications tend to take a kind of overkill approach. They target a vast array of symptoms, not all of which an allergy-sufferer may be experiencing. What's more, they suppress the symptoms, potentially causing a "backlash" problem later on, e.g., nasal passages that become more stuffed after clearing temporarily.

Homeopathic remedies for allergies are both gentle and specific (sometimes the specificity has to do with a particular symptom; sometimes with the particular allergen that is causing a reaction in the allergy sufferer).

Some homeopathic allergy remedies mentioned in this book are:

Allium cepa (the "red onion" remedy that works so well on a runny nose with clear discharge)

Ambrosia (the "ragweed" remedy, often very effective in the autumn when the ragweed count is high)

Apis (for hives and skin eruptions; for reactions to bee stings, shellfish, and strawberries)

Euphrasia (for allergy symptoms affecting the eyes)

Pulsitilla (for allergy-related sinusitus; sometimes works well on noses alternately runny and stuffy)

While all of the above can deal with occasional acute allergy symptoms quite nicely, perhaps the greatest advantage of homeopathy over allopathy when it comes to allergies is that someone with chronic allergies may actually get rid of their allergies altogether, or diminish them dramatically, by working under the guidance of a skilled homeopath over time. Again, this will be because the body's underlying imbalance—which is what causes it to overreact defensively to certain substances in the first place—will be corrected. (Since chronic allergies may predispose some children to asthma, working with a professional homeopath in this fashion is something you may seriously wish to consider.)

You may be thinking, what about allergy shots? If I just get them yearly, I'm fine. That may be true, but they still don't provide a permanent cure. And many parents do not like the idea of subjecting their children to this sort of yearly regime. (By the way, it is true that allergy shots do follow a principle of similars, in that they contain some of the original allergen that is causing the problem—but homeopathy works with much smaller doses, and is gentler all around.)

Some people worry that if they switch to homeopathy, they will have to go "cold turkey" on other kinds of allergy medication. But I have known many people who regularly use homeopathy but take those "big gun" allopathic medications every now and again. There are no known drug interactions that occur from mixing homeopathic remedies with other medications. And if a "mix and match" approach is most comfortable for you, especially at the beginning, no Homeopathy Police are going to ring your doorbell and tell you that you can't do it.

Flu

Flu shots, anyone? I don't know about you, but whenever I've taken them, I come down with the flu that season. I prefer to let my immune system do its job, with a little help from the remedies.

Some flu remedies I have mentioned are:

Gelsemium (good for shortening the length and severity of flu, especially when the symptoms include chills and a high level of fatigue)

Oscillococcinum® (a patented Boiron remedy that is also excellent for shortening the length of flu, and which I have known to virtually fend it off if taken at the first twinges)

In lieu of flu shots, you may also wish to discuss with your homeopathic practitioner using one of the above remedies in a preventative fashion before flu season begins.

Tummy Troubles

For routine tummy troubles (as opposed to those that are flu related), there are over-the-counter antacids. These usually contain substances such as magnesia or sodium bicarbonate which work (as the term "antacid" indicates) by counteracting stomach acid. These seem harmless enough, but in my experience the right homeopathic remedy can work more quickly and effectively than even a "plop, plop, fizz, fizz."

Among the remedies for indigestion, bloating, etc., are:

Carbo vegetalis (especially good for flatulence—the "etc." part of indigestion)

Nux vomica (especially handy if you've overindulged in rich foods)

And don't forget:

Argentum nitricum (for infant tummy woes that cause colic)

Diarrhea and Constipation—The Poop Group

Take a typical over-the-counter for diarrhea and what does it do? Plug you up, maybe for days on end. Take a laxative for constipation and, well, look out! There better not be anyone else in your family needing to use the bathroom.

As with so many allopathic medications, those for diarrhea and constipation treat a symptom by inducing the opposite symptom. By now, I bet you know what I am going to say next. Right: Homeopathy does not work that way.

Besides, homeopathy recognizes that there are different kinds of diarrhea and different causes. Among the diarrhea remedies are:

Argentum nitricum (for the loose bowels that accompany a state of anticipatory anxiety)
Arsenicum (especially for "traveler's diarrhea" that comes from food poisoning or drinking the water when one shouldn't)
Veratrum album (for diarrhea accompanying a stomach virus)
Podophyllum (good for kids whose bowel movements are preceded by loud rumbles; also good for diarrhea associated with teething)

Among those for constipation:

Alumina (especially good for cases where the person seems to be straining a great deal, with little or no result)

Lycopodium (for traveler's constipation)

Nux vomica (for constipation from indigestion; for children who are not having bowel movements but have not reached the uncomfortable "straining" stage yet; and—last but not least—for the kind of constipation that results from taking too many laxatives)

The Eyes Have It

Contact lens wearers of the world, unite (along with anyone else who suffers from eye irritation)! Have you ever really found a conventional over-the-counter eye drop (or a prescription one, for that matter) that actually makes you feel better—as opposed to one that seems to sting and burn, and only makes your condition worse? If you have, my hat's off to you. But I never did until I tried homeopathy.

Among the homeopathic eye remedies that are especially helpful:

Euphrasia (especially for eye stinging, burning, and itching that stems from allergy)

Nat mur (for dry eyes that need to produce more tears)

Optique® (an all-around eye drop from Boiron that brings sweet instant relief)

Infant Woes: Teething and Colic

The first remedy I mentioned in this book—the one that first exposed me to the wonders of homeopathy—was *chamomilla*. You already know this remedy can work like a charm to soothe a teething infant (and, by extension, that infant's frazzled parents).

What, by contrast, do conventional over-the-counter medications offer? Well, we can put a gel on our baby's gums, but many infants do not seem too pleased with that strategy—and any relief brought by it is only fleeting. We can also treat accompanying discomfort with acetaminophen. But we don't want to give too much of that, as we have been alerted that it can be dangerous.

Besides, by giving *chamomilla* we can offer one deep-acting, effective solution. The *chamomilla* not only eases the physical symptoms of teething—i.e., the aches, the drooling, the flushed cheeks—but deals with the whole constellation of emotional issues that accompany the trauma that you can imagine a baby experiences when its own body seems to be "turning against itself" by producing these odd pointy, spiky things that protrude from its soft, smooth gums.

While on the subject of infants, when it comes to colic, conventional medicine gives us . . . well, pretty much nothing. So what harm can come (and what good might!) from trying these homeopathic remedies?

Argentum nitricum (the most popular all-around colic remedy that deals with the baby's anxiety as well as physical discomforts)
Chamomilla (a good backup, especially when the baby won't let you put him down, or seems overtired but cannot sleep)
Lycopodium (when the condition is worse between 4 P.M. and 8 P.M.)

There are several combination baby colic remedies on the market as well, and you may wish to give these a try.

Sunburn and Skin Conditions

When we are sunburned, we tend to apply a soothing cream or lotion. There's nothing wrong with that, to be sure. Even homeopathic manufacturers offer us various soothing external preparations, in the form of creams and ointments made from *calendula*.

But one can also treat a sunburn, or other minor skin chaffings, irritations, and abrasions from the inside out, by taking *calendula* internally—that is, by taking pellets of the *calendula* remedy. This actually speeds a resolution of the condition, as opposed to simply offering temporary relief.

One of the reasons I bring this up (other than the fact that sunburn is such a common condition, despite moms' valiant attempts to slather their kids with sunscreen) is that homeopathy can also effectively treat other skin conditions—e.g., eczema, psoriasis, ringworm—from the inside out. And according to homeopathic principles, this is the best way to go about it.

Why? Because the skin is the outermost place (and hence, the most harmless way) that the body can express signs of an underlying imbalance.

If someone in your family has a chronic skin condition, you may be tempted to treat it with creams that contain steroids. These may suppress outward signs of the condition, and you may think, "Well, that's that." But alas, that may not be all there is to it. If the latent problem isn't addressed, it may be forced to "express itself" on a deeper level—creating more serious symptoms which will be harder to clear up in the long run.

I am not listing any particular homeopathic treatments for chronic skin conditions here, because these take some time to resolve and should be treated by a homeopath. But I did want to mention homeopathy's very sensible emphasis on the importance of recognizing such states for what they are—a message from the body that something is a bit off kilter.

Now that you know many of the ins and outs of homeopathy, along with some treatments for common conditions, you are equipped to begin dabbling and experimenting a bit. Or are you?

Actually, my guess is that right about now you have two fears. The first is that, despite all you've learned, homeopathy might not work for you.

I contend that if you are willing to stick with it, avail yourself of resources, do a little homework, and consult a professional when appropriate, chances are it will work very well.

The second fear, however, is more difficult to assuage. Perhaps, like many Medicine Moms before you, you are afraid homeopathy *will* work. Because if it does, that will open a whole new can of worms.

For instance, how much will you tell your conventional doctor; and how will you cover costs not on your conventional medical insurance plan? These practical concerns are completely reasonable, given the realities of our world and our health care system, and they are what the next chapters are all about.

CHAPTER

7

The Best of Both Worlds

Alternative no longer needs to mean one or the other. There should be no alternative other than the best health care known to man.
　　　　—Actress Jane Seymour, in testimony before
　　　　　the House Committee on Government Reform
　　　　　Hearing on Alternative Medicine

If we lived in France, certain things would be different. The croissants would be flakier, the fashions more chic, sure—but that's not the half of it. In France, we would find that homeopathy is part of everyday life. And perhaps what is most remarkable about it is how unremarkably it is regarded.

For one out of three Frenchmen, homeopathy is used all the time for everyday ailments. This, of course, includes French mothers and their *enfants*. In this part of the world, even young children quickly get the hang of twisting the cap of a little remedy tube so that the right number of pellets pop out as required.

Doing It French Style

Homeopathy's popularity from Paris to Lyon to Marseille, and points in between, is widely due to how many doctors readily accept what they call this *medicin douce* ("gentle medicine") and use it routinely in their practices. Oddly enough—at least from an American perspective, in which so many aspects of health care are segmented and specialized—in France, there is no such thing as a "homeopath" or a "naturopath." The physicians who prescribe homeopathic remedies use it alongside conventional medications, and in many instances will try it before anything else because they know it is efficient, natural, and safe. (Even the physician for the French national soccer team administers homeopathic remedies, such as *arnica* and flu-fighting *"Oscillo"* to his players.)

In America, this kind of model is an ideal we can hope for in the future. For now, being feisty, upstart Yanks, we are building our homeopathic resurgence primarily from a grass-roots mode. But if one looks closer, one can see that as our movement grows, that future is getting closer every day.

Homeopathy American Style: A Work in Progress

In September 1998, the results of a random telephone survey were revealed at a Stanford conference of doctors and other health care professionals. According to this poll, a whopping 69 percent of the respondents had used some form of complementary or alternative medicine in the preceding year.[1]

Who were they? As many demographic breakdowns show, it is likely they spanned three generations.

Seniors are increasingly attracted to alternative health models since older adults often have chronic conditions from which traditional medicine has not given them much relief. Baby boomers, highly health conscious, are always willing to experiment with the new (or actually in this case, the old, as many alternative therapies, including homeopathy, have been around for quite some time). The generation currently in their twenties and thirties, who value self-sufficiency, are also jumping on the alternative health care bandwagon.

Yet there are two very interesting facts about the individuals who are active consumers of alternative therapies. The first is that they are by no means willing to disregard the many benefits of conventional medicine. (Indeed, the respondents in the Stanford survey who used alternative methods had also seen conventional doctors on the average of four times yearly.) They are, by and large, thoughtful, well-rounded, and knowledgeable individuals who do not need to be convinced that conventional medicine has many treatments and procedures of obvious benefit in treating certain serious diseases and life-threatening conditions. Though they might supplement conventional treatments for such things with alternative therapies, they are hardly going to disregard convention altogether.

Ironically, however, the second interesting fact about alternative health care devotees is that they frequently do not inform their conventional physicians that they are also pursuing alternative care, whether by self-treating or by consulting with another practitioner. In its sweeping survey of alternative medicine trends in the 1990s, the *Journal of the American Medical Association* concluded that by 1997 less than 40 percent of all alternative therapies were being disclosed to physicians (it termed this a "don't ask and don't tell" policy).[2]

Patients and Doctors "In the Closet"

Now why in the world would anyone who is concerned enough with their own well-being and savvy enough to seek out alternative treatments neglect to share this information with their conventional practitioner?

I've never seen a study that asked respondents this particular question, so I asked some Medicine Moms. And I'll bet you can guess what the overwhelming answer was among parents who had not told their doctors (or their kids' pediatricians) about their interest in homeopathy.

Yes, you guessed it: fear. Fear of ridicule, fear of reprisal (as in expecting the doctor to say, "Get out of my office, you lunatic!"), and even fear of insulting or offending the doctors (by appearing to consider them less than omnipotent) were all given as reasons why doctors were allowed to remain in the dark.

Are some of these fears well founded? I'd be lying if I said no. Sure, I've heard of cases where conventional M.D.s belittled or pooh-poohed patients who sought any kind of care not strictly traditional. (Early on, I had such an experience.) I've even heard of a gauntlet or two thrown down—as in "You can't see me if you're going to do that voodoo."

Let's face it: Some of the men and women who have survived the grueling rites necessary to become a physician may be at least momentarily taken aback at having their authority appear to be challenged. And they may react defensively.

But if any of these things happen to you, rest assured that you—and your doctor—will survive. Besides, none of these scenarios is a foregone conclusion. If you were to come out of the closet and confess your interest in homeopathy (or any other alternative treatment) to your family physician, you might be pleasantly surprised. Because, amazingly enough, some of them—not all, but some—are in the closet as well!

For example, here is what one Medicine Mom told me happened to her when she finally divulged her little secret to her daughter's pediatrician:

On several occasions, my daughter had been prescribed an antibiotic for ear infection which I did not use. Instead I treated her with homeopathic remedies. I would religiously go back to the doctor two weeks after she'd been diagnosed to make sure her condition had cleared up. It always had. After about the third time this happened over the course of a year and a half, I said to the doctor, "Look, I'm kind of scared to tell you this, but I really don't believe in antibiotics for ear infections, and I haven't been using them, but as you can see it's all worked out fine." I saw his eyes widen for a minute, then he said, "I agree with you. They're given out way too much." I just about fell off my chair. Then he wanted to know what I had been doing instead, and he said he knew a little bit about homeopathy and was planning to learn more about it, along with some other things.

You know I was so happy and stunned I sort of lost my bearings and didn't ask him anything else right then. But now I really would like to know, if this was the way he felt, how come he never told me before?

As astonishing as it seems, I have heard a number of similar stories. Some physicians actually seem relieved when Medicine Moms come clean, and some take the occasion to confess their own interest in integrative medicine.

But the question the similarly relieved moms seem to end up with is: *Why did the doctor wait for me to bring it up?*

Odds are some of the reasons have to do with formalities and some with legalities. What I mean by formalities has to do with the way our conventional health care system works. If you are a typical American "health care consumer," chances are you don't generally spend very much time one-on-one with your own doctor, let alone your kids' doctor. You don't really know much about them, and they in turn know very little about you—unless you make it a point to tell them. When any two people don't know a lot about each other, it follows that a lot of assumptions are made. In the cases of doctors and patients, each party probably assumes that the other is more interested in status quo medical interventions than anything else.

As far as legalities, alas we again have to face the reality that America's legal system is such that many practitioners are reticent about going out on anything that might be considered a limb. Some physicians fear that to offer alternatives to traditional allopathy may put them at greater risk for potential patient legal claims—and not necessarily because they fear the therapies are harmful but because, as we already know, there is legal safety in sticking with the norm.

This may sound a tad cowardly on doctors' parts, but don't be too hasty to judge. Consider that even a frivolous claim or litigation may sometimes be enough to send one's malpractice insurance premiums sky high, and wreak havoc with one's career. You, too, might be excessively cautious under the circumstances.

The good news is that, with luck, some of this self-protective reticence to recommend alternatives may soon begin to wane. Ironically, the *Journal of the American Medical Association* reports that there are fewer malpractice claims against so-called alternative practitioners than there are against conventional physicians.[3]

Besides, as more and more of us express an interest in alternative care, "going out on a limb" may not seem so legally daunting. This, quite simply, is because that limb is becoming more and more populated. Should we edge closer to the French-style medical system, where a high percentage of doctors consider homeopathy a routine intervention, then there will be a new standard of what, exactly, falls within the norm.

Let's face it, not all of our doctors will be receptive to our forays into homeopathy, even as an adjunct to allopathic medicine. But on balance, it's a good idea to broach the subject. It's really not fair to doctors or patients when physicians don't know what their customers are doing outside of the consultation room. Your doctor may not be Patch Adams, but he just might be more open-minded than you think. Or you may serve to open his mind, even a chink, paving the way for other Medicine Moms to follow.

Of course, whenever you tell someone something unexpected, their reaction can depend a lot on *how* you tell them. No one wants to feel sand-bagged. And just as you do not want to feel belittled or dismissed by your doctor, neither does he want to be made to feel that way by you. With that in mind, I have compiled from a group of Medicine Moms what they consider to be an effective list of guidelines for "coming out of the closet" to your conventional physician in a manner that may prove beneficial to you both.

Building a Bridge to Your Physician

- Using the term "complementary" or "integrative" medicine (which tends to be less threatening than "alternative"), start with a few exploratory feeler questions. You can try asking your physician if he has any interest in this, or has ever been curious about it, or even how he would react to a patient who wanted to try such-and-such a treatment. If you don't hit a stone wall, you can go on from there. (If you do hit a stone wall, please read the next section of this chapter before banging your head against it.)

- In a discussion, have your facts at hand. This will give you confidence and show that you are serious, and it will also help you keep your doctor from getting off track. For example, some doctors may think you are referring to herbs when you start to talk about homeopathy and may launch into a lecture on the dangers of herbs. If you can quickly explain the difference between the two modalities (remember, homeopathy uses infinitesimal doses and the Law of Similars), you can head this sort of thing off at the pass.

- Notice that the above guideline contains the word "quickly." Alas, the reality of modern conventional medicine is such that you are not likely going to be allotted a great deal of time to make your points. You'll likelier win an ally—or at least not alienate a skeptic—if you are brief and to the point. Also, take a breath once in a while and give your doctor a chance to respond or ask questions. Sometimes when we are nervous and we finally start to blurt something out, we can't seem to come up for air.

- Be clear about your personal preferences. As physician Mary Ann Block wrote in her book, *No More Amoxicillin,* "I was told many times during my medical training that the patient wants a prescription when he visits the doctor's office, and if he doesn't get one, he will find another doctor who will prescribe one."[4] Don't give your physician the chance to make this assumption if it's not what you want.

- Let your doctor know he has your "informed consent" to use nonallopathic means to address your or your child's ailment or, as the case may be, to refer you to a practitioner more familiar with complementary medicine. "Informed consent" is a phrase that signals to him you are not likely to turn around and accuse him of wrongdoing later on for not doing the routine thing. I know one Medicine Mom who, along with her practitioner, has developed a "code" wherein he tells her that "for the record" he is recommending such-and-such, though she may choose to do otherwise. She replies that "for the record" she understands. Then she goes ahead and uses homeopathy, and all parties are relatively content.

What if My Doctor Is Unreceptive?

The mom who uses this "for the record" phrase confided she looked forward to a day when she and her physician could have more of an open dialogue, and share their resources. But while she aspires to that ideal, in the meanwhile she does the best she can.

Things being what they are—and by "things" I mean insurance plans, geographical limitations, economics, and the like—not all of us have the luxury of finding what we might consider the ideal, open-minded doctor. Sometimes we do have to find a way to tiptoe through a system that all parties would probably agree is less than perfect.

Indeed, sometimes we do hit the aforementioned stone wall, and may be faced with the unhappy choice of either shopping around for another practitioner (not always simple, given insurance restrictions) or remaining "closeted." (No one ever said life was fair!) In such a case—if there is any way possible to do so—finding a more simpatico physician is a far safer, sensible, and more constructive choice than the latter course of action.

But this may well bring you to the next obvious question—money. Suppose finding another practitioner means "going out of network," as they say, to a practitioner whose visits are not as fully covered (or maybe not covered at all) by insurance benefits? Suppose you have to drive farther to visit a more open-minded doctor? And while we're on the subject, suppose that—ironically enough—expensive antibiotics and other prescription drugs are covered by your health care plan while homeopathic remedies are not?

Is it worth all the expense, let alone all the hassle?

That is the subject of the next chapter. And though the subject of money can cause some of us to get our stomachs knotted in advance, I urge you to relax. For on the whole, there is much good news ahead.

CHAPTER
8

What's It Going to Cost Me?

Better see rightly on a pound a week than squint on a million.

—George Bernard Shaw

Change is not without inconvenience, even from worse to better.

—Richard Hooker, English theologian

As we already know, a majority of American medical schools are adding courses on complementary and alternative medicine to their curriculum, and medical students are expressing a strong interest in taking them. In addition, hospitals are adding complementary medical centers to their facilities, and they are advertising them aggressively. Why is all this happening? Of course, in part, it is because there is a growing belief that Western medicine can be greatly enhanced and expanded upon by incorporating other systems. But it is also, in part, because of the bottom line.

Conservatively estimated, total consumer expenditures on alternative therapies in the late 1990s exceeded $20 billion annually.[1] And by all accounts, that figure is now rapidly approaching $30 billion. By anyone's standards, this is a large chunk of change. Businesses and institutions cannot help but want a part of it for themselves, and—three cheers for the profit motive!—this will benefit all of us who are interested in nonconventional medicine.

The health care industry is, slowly but surely, turning into a buyer's market. And as Medicine Moms, we are voting with our dollars to speed that process along.

The "Out-of-Pocket" Phenomenon

For the time being, much of the money being spent on alternative therapies is coming out of the pockets (or pocketbooks, as the case may be) of the individuals who desire such services. Indeed, the majority of people who sought such services over the last decade parted with their own hard-earned dollars in order to do so.[2]

When you consider that, over the same period of time, consumers paid less of their own conventional health care costs (government and private insurers bore more of the brunt[3]), the out-of-pocket trend for alternative care is really quite noteworthy. What it indicates is that despite a system which, in general, financially rewards people for staying inside the box, people are exploring outside the box in droves.

Does this mean that money is no object to such people? Does it mean that alternative care in America is strictly a luxury for the very affluent? I've heard that said, and perhaps years ago it was substantially true. But from what I have seen of late, that is no longer the case.

All around me, I see people with a wide range of income levels biting the financial bullet. They are coming up with whatever resources they have to if they feel strongly that the well-being of their family is at stake.

What, exactly, it may cost any one of us to pursue homeopathic treatment will vary. You may get lucky and find an M.D. or D.O. who incorporates homeopathy into his practice and is, in whole or in part, covered by your insurance plan. But then again, you may not be so blessed. Depending on your coverage, you may be very limited in your choice of practitioners. And while using homeopathic remedies themselves may not stretch your budget (the cost for a vial of 75 or so medicinal pellets tends to run between $5 and $6), the thought of consulting a homeopath on your own dime can, at first, seem daunting.

Remember, the initial consultation with a homeopath takes quite some time due to its in-depth nature. Because of this, a first visit can run upwards of $150 (keep in mind you will likely get at least an hour of the practitioner's time, as opposed to the conventional ten minutes). Subsequent visits tend to be far less costly, and once you know more about homeopathy yourself, you may be satisfied with office visits spaced farther apart. Still, it's easy to appreciate why someone who is used to a "ten-dollar copayment" for a doctor's appointment might question their sanity when they find themselves digging deep into their own cookie jar for a fistful of cash.

Still, more and more of us are doing it, for we understand there are many ways in which to figure "cost."

Let me ask you a few questions:

- How many days of school and work do your family members miss each year because of flu, colds, allergies, ear infections, and the like?
- How much time do you spend sitting in the waiting room of a pediatrician's office (let alone trying to get through on the phone)?
- After all that, how much time do you get to spend with the pediatrician?
- What is the "cost" of the stress you endure seeing your kids come down with the same ailments over and over again?
- What "price" can you put on good health, and on gaining a greater degree of control over your family's overall well-being?

When you add up all the factors involved and view the big picture, it's easy to see why so many people are making the decision to spend their own money on homeopathy. But now, here's the really encouraging part. What we spend today sends a message to insurance companies as to *what we value.* And since insurance companies want customers, as all businesses do, they can't help but pay attention.

This adds more fuel to an already burning fire. For the truth is that homeopathy has already gained the attention of all parties involved in health care oversight, including not just insurance companies, but private employers and government.

That is because these institutions are learning—as many individuals already have—the many ways in which homeopathy makes sound financial sense.

It's Cost-Effective!

In 1991, a study conducted by the French government found that the annual cost to France's social security system for patients using the services of a homeopathic physician was 15 percent less than those using conventional physicians. The savings amount was attributed to the reduction in costs of diagnostic tests and to the lower cost of homeopathic medicines. [4] This study got a great deal of media play. And why wouldn't it, in an era where everyone is concerned with the seeming impossibility of keeping up with health care costs?

Here at home, government seems to have gotten wind of the situation. The state of Maryland, for instance, appointed a commission in 1995 to study complementary forms of health care. And the commission found that in the areas studied, complementary therapies were equally if not more effective than traditional methods and—here it comes—came in at only a fraction of the cost.[5] Suddenly, it seems government has a good reason to pay more attention to CAM than it ever has before.

Now here's more fascinating news from Europe. In 1996, an additional French study confirmed the results of the 1991 survey. It also added that the number of paid sick leave days by patients under the care of homeopathic physicians was 3. 5 times less than patients under the care of conventional general practitioners.[6] Were I an employer, I know I would surely find this a grabber.

Indeed, a growing number of American employers are now beginning to evaluate the benefits of offering alternative treatments, including homeopathy, in their benefits package. It is one way to increase productivity and enhance continuity on the job. Better yet, it is, in the words of Darrell Askey, CFO of Celestial Seasonings (one of the many companies participating in this trend) a "way to foster employee morale."[7] In and of itself, this is a key ingredient of any successful business.

As for insurers, they, too, tend to know a good thing when they see it. From their perspective, CAM treatments, including homeopathy, are beginning to look very intriguing. Not surprisingly, they've done some cost studies of their own. One of these, a pilot conducted by Blue Cross/Blue Shield's Alternapath program, showed decreased visits per patient and an overall reduction in costs when patients utilize alternative care practitioners—and this is *despite* the fact that the costs of initial consultations may be relatively high.[8]

What's more, covering CAM will allow insurers to become more competitive in the marketplace by meeting a swelling consumer demand. In a study funded by the National Institute of Health's Office of Alternative Medicine, 56 percent of respondents said they wanted their health care plan to cover complementary and alternative therapies, and a recent study by Landmark Healthcare placed that number at 79 percent.[9]

At the time of this writing, more and more insurers are incorporating alternative health care benefits—which cover everything from massage therapy and nutritional counseling to acupuncture and, yes, homeopathy—into some of their plans. These insurers include such giants as Blue Cross (in North Carolina, Washington, Alaska, and California), California Pacific, HealthNet, Kaiser Permanente, Mutual of Omaha, Oxford, and Prudential (though, obviously, if you are insured by any of these good folks, you will need to check the specific benefits in your individual policy).

As incredible as it may seem, the managed care system, for all its inherent difficulties, may well exhibit a saving grace. For the most practical of reasons—cost effectiveness and competitiveness—it is likely to emerge as one of the chief advocating forces of homeopathy in this country.

What's Taking So Long?

Of course, when it's your child who wakes up in the middle of the night with yet another ear infection and you are at the end of your rope, it really isn't all that immediately comforting to know that probably one day your health plan will cover homeopathy. If you're still among the many Medicine Moms who will have to pay part or all of your costs for homeopathic treatment out of pocket for now, here's why: Many insurers still want to see more academically proven scientific research on homeopathy.

Such studies take time—and money. But an increasing number of them are on the horizon. The more interested consumers become in homeopathy, the more academia, drug companies, and government-funded agencies are willing to invest in researching it. Undoubtedly the studies that are coming will be bigger and better than any done in the past. With more resources available, larger population samples can be used, and follow-ups can be more long-term. Best of all, methodology can be improved, and ideally, the results of these studies will be based not just on patients being treated with generalized remedies (e.g., *Allium cepa* or *ambrosia* for hayfever) but with remedies tailored to their individual symptoms by a professional homeopath.

Those of us who have seen homeopathy at work are thrilled at such prospects. We know how well homeopathy has fared in studies up until now, and we also know that the more rigorous the study, the better homeopathy proves out.

So, if you are one of those who are still patiently (or impatiently) waiting for your health coverage to catch up with the twenty-first century, remember this mantra: Bring on the scientists!

Why Everyone Will Benefit

Will *everyone* begin to incorporate homeopathy into their health regime early in this century? Of course not. But in a world with many options, this will increasingly be a viable one. Happily, such a trend will benefit virtually everyone—even those who do not personally choose to use homeopathy.

Here's how:

- Right now, tens of millions of workdays each year are lost to flu, colds, allergies, and related ailments. Given how homeopathy can shorten the course and lessen the severity of such conditions, overall workplace productivity—hence the gross national product—should rise.
- Right now billions are spent annually to treat these same ailments (plus billions more on your kids' ear infections). These figures will drop dramatically, freeing resources for other critical medical purposes.
- Visits to emergency rooms—an enormous burden on the health care system, and costly for everyone in the end—will also be curtailed.
- Antibiotics abuse, universally acknowledged as a grave danger to us all, will subside—allowing these powerful drugs to work best when you or your kids *really* need them most.
- The chronic conditions of a growing population of elders will be more gently—and less expensively—treated.
- Lower income families will be able to avail themselves of safe, effective homeopathic services at subsidized clinics at a fraction of the cost of what such facilities now cost. (And there will be more private "alternative" practitioners able to donate *pro bono* time in their own practices.)
- Last, but not least, the environment will benefit, as manufacturing homeopathic remedies requires only the smallest amount of natural resources.

Individual Responsibility: What Will You Choose?

Of course, none of this is going to happen magically. In the final analysis, all "movements" in society consist of nothing more than a series of choices made by individuals. We are, each of us, responsible for ourselves and the world we live in. Knowing that, if you want your health plan to provide coverage for complementary treatments such as homeopathy, you still may have to ante up in a certain way.

At the end of World War II, companies desperate to attract workers offered health benefits as an incentive. In ensuing decades, the American public came to take such arrangements more or less for granted. But in recent years, as many of us are already keenly aware, this trend has been reversing itself. Employers are more reluctant to foot an employee's entire health care bill, and the portion workers are asked to contribute each year from their paychecks is ever on the rise. Couple this phenomenon with the swelling ranks of self-employed freelancers and entrepreneurs, and what it all adds up to is the fact that more and more of us are going to be choosing—and paying for—more and more of our own health care insurance anyhow.

Often, when we are asked to choose our own health care plans based on price tag, we look primarily at the bottom line—and in a short-sighted way. If—or rather, when—you need to make such choices, it pays (and I mean that literally) to make certain you are a thoroughly educated consumer.

Some things Medicine Moms are already doing, and which you can do as well:

- Factor in not just the overt "cost," but look deeper at the many real savings your family will incur by selecting coverage that includes CAM (e.g., savings of time, long-term savings of money, savings of angst, and of sleepless nights spent tending sick, unhappy kids).
- Explore supplementary health care policies which cover CAM benefits your primary policy may not. (More of these are cropping up every day, and searching for them on the World Wide Web is really the best way to keep up.)
- Investigate tax-free medical reimbursement accounts, sometimes available as payroll deductions. With this money you

can pay for services your regular insurance won't cover by using tax-free dollars set aside for this purpose. (But be careful of the "use it or lose it" feature where you forfeit any dollars not spent in the calendar year.)

- Join the push for legislation for tax-free medical savings accounts, with which individuals will be able to purchase discretionary medical services that best meet their needs. (Some proposals suggest that any unused sums be allowed to be rolled over into IRAs.) Again, the Internet is a wonderful way to keep up with developments in this area.

I don't mean to give the impression that pursuing homeopathy, in its medicinal aspects and its financial ones, needs to be your full-time vocation. Actually, it will enhance your life and free up time, overall. But some initial effort is time well spent.

The short-term investment of effort and, yes, money you make today will lead to profound benefits in the long run. For ultimately, homeopathy itself is a frugal system of medicine—one that manages to do so very much with so very little. That "less is more" philosophy incorporates the kind of enlightened frugality that gives rise to abundance for all.

CHAPTER

9

Where Do We Go from Here?

Needs, passions and interests are the sole spring of actions.
—Georg Hegel, German philosopher

If you've read this far along in *Medicine Moms,* perhaps by now you and your family have at least dabbled in some homeopathic healing. If so, here are some of the things that have likely happened:

- You have stopped panicking at, and overreacting to, the slightest symptoms of ailments such as colds and earaches.
- You are more confident and calmer in dealing with all medical matters, as you are armed with information, or know where to find it.
- You have reduced your use of over-the-counter suppressive medications—those antihistamines, decongestants, cough suppressants, and antifebrile drugs you used to rely on so often—and have found that they have migrated to the back of your medicine cabinet, while gentle homeopathic remedies have shifted front and center.
- You have reduced your use of prescription antibiotics.
- You are not fighting with your kids about "taking their medicine" the way you used to.
- Your family, while still succumbing to life's little illnesses, is enduring milder cases of them for shorter periods of time—because your immune systems are being allowed to do their jobs.

This all seems pretty good, doesn't it? But in fact, if you are interested in taking the next step, things may soon get even better.

As helpful as it is to use homeopathy to treat commonly occurring acute illnesses, there is another level to which it can be taken. In consultation with a professional, you may want to look into constitutional remedies.

What Is a "Constitutional"?

A constitutional remedy is a not a "medication" in the way traditional allopathy uses the term, in that it isn't something given to counteract a symptom. It is also not the same as the remedies one might give homeopathically to promote quicker healing of a self-limiting condition. It is, instead, a preventative remedy, meant to strengthen an individual overall, alleviate chronic conditions, and keep repetitive acute illnesses from recurring.

In general, constitutional remedies are not given while someone is in the grips of an acute illness. They are given when active symptoms of any such illness have subsided. For it is then that a homeopath can get a picture of how a patient appears, acts, and feels—both physically and emotionally—in his or her everyday state.

Constitutionals are prescribed based on a full and complete picture of an individual, a kind of physiopsychological gestalt. Indeed, one of the reasons homeopaths ask so many detailed—and sometimes seemingly irrelevant—questions during an initial interview is that they are attempting to begin to get a sense of what constitutional "type" a patient might be.

In medical systems other than Western allopathy, the idea that we all fall into a particular classification that predisposes us to certain strengths and weaknesses is quite common—and very useful in terms of prescribing. In homeopathy, the nomenclature of these constitutional types corresponds to the remedy they most need to bring them into balance and nudge them in the direction of total well-being.

Thus, a homeopath may say you are a Phosphorus type, or that your child is, perhaps, a Pulsitilla. Of course if you are anything like me and most other Medicine Moms, you will immediately ask if these are "good things" or "bad things" to be.

Well, let me save you some anxiety. Finding out your constitutional type is not like getting a grade on a report card. It is a kind of shorthand for summing up the tendencies of your mind-body complex. It allows your homeopath to discover the best individualized overall remedy for you (hence a Phosphorus type will be treated with *phosphorus,* a Pulsitilla with *pulsitilla*).

Each of us is, in fact, a product of all our input and experiences. This includes our genetic makeup and any congenital conditions, our body type and metabolism, environmental influences, our emotional high points and traumas, our disposition and attitudes, our way of relating to others, and our habits, preferences, and peccadilloes. The constitutional remedy is meant to pinpoint and correct any elements in this mix that result in vulnerabilities to certain kinds of stress. In short, they target whatever your particular "Achilles' heel" may be.

Why do this? Because not to do it—to go on treating only symptomatic conditions as they arise—would be, as my own homeopathic physician put it, "to treat the branches of a tree, without treating its roots." Yes, treating the branches is useful, but dig deeper and the entire organism can really flourish from the ground up—or in the case of people, a more exact metaphor would be *from the inside out.*

What Is a Constitutional Dose?

A constitutional is not given the same way as acute medications, nor is it given in the same dosages. Depending on how your homeopath works, it will most likely be given in a very high potency (e.g., a 10M—M standing for a thousand dilutions), or in what's called an LM potency (the LM is a preparation method discovered by Hahnemann which combines the effectiveness of high-strength dosages with the gentleness of low-strength dosages). How often it will be given depends on the individual case.

But the most important thing you need to know about the constitutional is that this is definitely one of those areas of homeopathy where you must rely on a professional. In other words, do not try this at home.

There are several good books about identifying your kids' constitutional types—or yours or your spouse's for that matter (I recommend a few of them in the Resources section). This is fun to do. But please stop short of actually giving them the remedy. Even if you do zero in on the one appropriate remedy out of many, and even if you can purchase the proper dosage strength (some mail order services will send them), there are simply too many variables for you to handle on your own. Let a homeopath take stock of the case, and determine how often the constitutional should be given, when it should be stopped—or changed, because the patient has changed— and so on.

What Might Result from a Constitutional?

If the right constitutional is given, the results—over time—can be amazing to behold. It's like hitting the bull's-eye of bull's-eyes. Overall the recipients will be healthier, heartier, and more resilient mentally and physically. They will probably contract acute illnesses far less often, and chronic conditions—which seemed to be an inexorable part of their lives—may begin to dissipate.

In the physical realm, I have seen many people—both adults and children—who suffered profusely with allergies their whole lives, begin to live free of dread about the pollen count. I have seen many kids go from having an ear infection every month or two to having one every year or two. (My own son, as I mentioned earlier, was one.) I have seen moms part with PMS on a permanent basis. And I even knew a woman suffering from hair loss whose condition was reversed after taking her constitutional.

On an emotional level, results may be even more significant. Many Medicine Moms have commented to me how overactive children have calmed down after taking their constitutionals, or how shy children have seemed to come out of their shells. One of them swears her son's constitutional got him to clean up his room—a feat she could never accomplish through nagging, threats or bribes.

To give you one example of how strongly a constitutional may affect a child on an emotional/developmental level, here is a brief excerpt from an e-mail correspondence I had with a Medicine Mom in England. This mother, whom I'll call Dinah, had taken her three-and-a-half-year-old son to a homeopath because of persistent urinary tract infections. The homeopath believed the urinary problems were due to a constitutional weakness and prescribed a constitutional forthwith. The urinary problems indeed cleared up. But to Dinah's surprise, she got more than she'd bargained for.

She wrote:

Anthony had always been distant, uncommunicative, and difficult to discipline . . . Since being given his remedy, he has become a sensitive, aware and sensible little boy.

Not all constitutionals will induce startling results, but it is surprising how often they smooth over the rough edges of the personality. When they do, especially in the case of children, they can do so quite rapidly. Remember, constitutionals work on vulnerabilities that result from everything our minds and bodies have experienced. To do this, they have to work on peeling through layers of physical and emotional stressors we have incorporated. Children, having lived fewer years than adults, simply have fewer layers that need peeling.

ADD and Homeopathy

The psychological/developmental benefits available to children through homeopathy have, as of late, resulted in some very promising research. Some researchers are hypothesizing that homeopathy can be an invaluable treatment tool for children with attention deficit disorder (ADD) and attention deficit hyperactivity disorder (ADHD). In one controlled study of forty-three children diagnosed with ADHD, those treated with an individually tailored homeopathic remedy—after having been previously treated with placebo—showed significant improvement.[1]

ADD and ADHD have become so pervasive that such developments are well worth following, especially when one considers that the conventional Ritalin® treatment used in many cases can potentially result in deleterious side effects from loss of appetite and sleeplessness to joint pain, chest pain, and irregular heartbeat. Interestingly, Ritalin® is a stimulant, and since it is used to treat children who are already inattentive and hyperactive, that makes it one of the relatively rare examples in allopathic pharmacology of treating a condition with a "similar." But just to be clear, Ritalin® and other stimulant drugs used to treat ADD and ADHD are not homeopathic in principle, as they do not adhere to the Law of the Minimum Dose. What's more, if you have a child who has been diagnosed ADD or ADHD and seek homeopathic treatment, that child will not be treated with one-size fits-all medication, but will be given a remedy—perhaps a constitutional—that fits his unique symptom picture.

Homeopathy and Other Psychological Conditions

Just as homeopathy can potentially be effective for kids with ADD and ADHD, some have found it effective for kids with other kinds of emotional or developmental problems, including impulse control and anger management difficulties (which may result in a diagnosis such as conduct disorder), post-traumatic stress syndrome (e.g., from the aftereffects of trauma or abuse), and so on.

Naturally, I am not suggesting that a visit to a homeopath, in and of itself, will necessarily result in the swift and total resolution of such complex problems. But homeopathy may be a valuable avenue to pursue as a complement to a variety of other approaches. And this holds true for the emotional problems of adults as well as children.

As a psychotherapist myself (my job when I am not wearing my mom hat), I have recently become very interested in combining psychotherapy and homeopathy. What's more, I have witnessed some remarkable success stories.

There was one woman, for example, who had suffered from insomnia for as long as she could remember. She was in her late thirties when I met her, and had already tried every sleep-inducing technique she'd ever heard of, to no avail. Together, we tried everything *I* could think of—from exploring the childhood nighttime fears she suspected contributed to the problem, to employing various self-hypnosis, relaxation, and meditation techniques. But we did not make much headway. She also consulted a psychopharmacologist, who gave up after he told her he had exhausted his entire arsenal of sleep-inducing medications, with no permanent improvement. Although I honestly didn't know if it would help, I suggested the client just might want to try consulting a homeopath, which she did. He prescribed *Aurum metallicum* (gold) in an LM potency as a constitutional, and within a couple of weeks she was actually—finally—getting a good night's sleep on a routine basis.

Since then, I have been more predisposed to recommending homeopathy as a complement to therapy when it seems appropriate. I have now seen *Natrum muriaticum* help certain people cope with unresolved feelings of sadness and loss (this remedy, you may recall, is sea salt, and among other things, it literally helps them shed tears long held back). And I have seen *Argentum nitricum* (silver nitrate) successfully used to help fend off panic attacks by people who do not feel comfortable using allopathic anxiety medications, which can easily be habit-forming.

I am by no means alone in my growing fascination with homeopathy's potential application to the field of mental health. In fact, a growing number of mental health professionals are becoming interested in exploring alternative medicines.

At first, most of this interest sprang from the sometimes successful use of such herbs as St. John's wort to treat depression and kava kava to treat anxiety. Yet homeopathy has the potential to be even more effective than herbs in this area, because of its individualized nature. Where herbology has one remedy for depression, homeopathy has dozens, and the one selected would ideally correspond to exactly how depression manifested itself in a particular person (e.g., some people overeat and oversleep when depressed; others can't eat or sleep much at all—differing symptom pictures and hence different remedies).

The homeopathic approach to mental health is just beginning to gain general notice, but the picture is promising. Even the American Psychiatric Association has recently begun including homeopathic seminars in its annual conference. Again, I ask you, can you get more mainstream than this?

Homeopathy and the Life Cycle

I suspect you picked up this book primarily because you were interested in the prospect of learning about homeopathy for children's common ailments. But as you've gone along you may, like many Medicine Moms before you, have come to realize you don't want to miss out on more of a good thing. And really, why should anyone?

As you proceed with your homeopathic interests, be they casual or more serious, you will no doubt trip across information concerning the many uses of homeopathy from one end of life to the other.

Homeopathic remedies, for example, can be useful for a postpartum mother and her newborn child; for the pubescent preteen and the maturing adolescent; for problems of infertility and menopause; for the elderly suffering chronic conditions (such as arthritis); and even for treatment of the terminally ill (where it can sometimes be used in conjunction with allopathic treatments to ease discomfort and enhance the quality of life that remains).

Your continued interest in homeopathy can be the catalyst for various members of your family—not just your young children, but your grown children, your spouse, your aging parents, and (last but, I hope, never least) yourself—to enjoy a healthier life in every sense.

Staying involved in homeopathy will be a way for you to remain alert to your own and your family's changing health profiles over the years. It will encourage you to pay attention to subtleties and nuances that might otherwise have slipped by undetected, until perhaps things had progressed too far. And it will allow you to exert a positive influence on all around you.

In keeping up your Medicine Momhood, you will stay connected—to yourself, to your loved ones, and to a growing community of like-minded people who share your concerns, your commitment, and your hopes.

EPILOGUE

A Classic Science in a Modern Era

It's the same each time with progress. First they ignore you, then they say you're mad, then dangerous, then there's a pause, and then you can't find anyone who disagrees with you.

—Tony Benn, British politician

Homeopathy is a classic science, founded some two centuries ago. Yet like so many world-altering ideas—the roundness of the earth, the location of the sun in the center of the solar system, the invention of the steam engine—it was in many ways presented ahead of its time.

Happily for us, this system of medicine is ideally suited for application in the Third Millennium. The reasons for this are many.

First, there is a profound need for homeopathy and its unique approach. Due to environmental and psychological stressors—and to the fact that we have spent so many years suppressing acute symptoms—chronic illnesses, which compromise the quality of life, are on the rise. Living longer than ever, we all want to feel better while doing it. And dissatisfied with our "assembly line" approach to health care, we are demanding a combination of evidence-based medicine and individualized, relationship-centered care.

Second, the zeitgeist, i.e., the attitude and atmosphere of the times, is open to it. Today, many of us are open to new ways of thinking, and will willingly consider paradigms that challenge the status quo. We have seen such radical changes in our lifetime, so many "modern miracles" if you will, that we are intrigued to entertain yet one more.

Third, and extremely important, homeopathy is finally being coupled with the information technology of which it is worthy. It's a happy and productive marriage.

Today, thanks to the Internet and the astounding level of communication it facilitates, anyone anywhere who has access to a computer (whether at home, at school, or in a public library), can tap into websites and into vast databases, learning a tremendous amount about homeopathy. They can obtain information about remedies, locate practitioners and suppliers, follow developing research, and—best of all—share what they have learned with people in virtually every corner of the earth. (One can, for example, post the symptoms of a local flu epidemic in one's town and the remedy that has been most helpful for it, potentially helping other communities in the process.) In short, the world is wired for homeopathy.

Now all that's required is your participation. Through your interest, and the interest of others like you and like me, Medicine Moms will thrive, while reclaiming the innate well-being of their families.

Relax, now. I am not advising you become an evangelist or begin a crusade. I know—trust me, no one knows better—you have ten thousand things on your plate. So now you have ten thousand and one. But, hey, the last one is a good one!

In the remaining pages of this book you will find an annotated resource section, along with a homeopathic glossary and a few other goodies to help you on your way.

Start small. Explore. Dabble. Think. Ask. And ask again. Let your curiosity, your questions, and your very good intentions toward the people you love most guide you to the medical technology of the future.

And enjoy it in the very best of health.

Resources for Medicine Moms

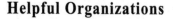

Helpful Organizations

NATIONAL CENTER FOR HOMEOPATHY (NCH)
801 North Fairfax Street
Suite 306
Alexandria, VA 22314
703-548-7790
703-548-7792 (fax)
Website: www.homeopathic.org

Every Medicine Mom could benefit from a yearly membership (which costs $40) to this highly user-friendly organization.

The NCH publishes a monthly magazine, *Homeopathy Today,* filled with all kinds of news, research updates, announcements of upcoming courses and events, etc., which is always a treat to find in one's mailbox. Better still, it publishes a yearly Membership Directory and Homeopathic Resource Guide, which one can use to locate like-minded folk in one's immediate area—as well as local practitioners. And if, in locating likeminded folk, you decide to form a study group, the NCH will furnish you with a wonderful *NCH Study Guide* to get you started.

The NCH sponsors summer courses (many over weekends, great fun if you can get your family to spare you for a few days) and a yearly national convention, which is well worth attending if you become more serious about your studies, or just want an interesting excursion. (By the way, you get a discount on all of this with membership, as well as on books and products.)

Visit the NCH website (you don't need to be a member) for a directory of practitioners, and to tap into a wonderful database of such things as "Homeopathy in the News" and "Homeopathy and the Law." You can access recent research studies and cost-effectiveness studies too.

The NCH has been a strong voice in the continued quest for increased access to homeopathic care for one and all. Once you get to know the organization, you may well want to add your voice to its chorus.

THE COUNCIL ON HOMEOPATHIC CERTIFICATION
(CHC)
1199 Sanchez
San Francisco, CA 94114
415-789-7677
415-695-8220 (fax)
Website: www.homeopathy-council.org/contact.htm

The mission of this organization is to set national education and certification standards for homeopaths from all the major health care professions, as well as for laypeople who train as professional homeopaths. Its greatest use for Medicine Moms can be in helping you find a qualified homeopath in your area. Visit their Website for a directory, and to learn about the rigorous standards which must be met for anyone to earn a CCH (Certified in Classical Homeopathy) credential.

HOMEOPATHIC ACADEMY OF NATUROPATHIC
PHYSICIANS (HANP)
12132 Foster Place
Portland, OR 97266
503-761-3298
Website: www.healthy.net/HANP

Naturopathic physicians (N.D.s), who generally integrate several alternate therapies—e.g., homeopathy, herbology, acupuncture, etc.—are licensed in about a dozen states. This organization's goal is to further N.D.s expertise in homeopathy. There is a searchable membership and practitioner database at their Website.

Informative Websites—Homeopathy

In addition to the Websites of the above organizations, the following Websites offer a plethora of information for inquiring Medicine Moms.

www.homeopathyhome.com

This is a truly comprehensive, and international, site. It has links to just about everything you'd ever want to find, including homeopathic organizations around the world, homeopathic pharmacies and hospitals, homeopathic veterinary services, remedy suppliers, etc. It also has a twenty-four-hour chat room and a discussion page where you can post questions and receive answers via e-mail from all over.

www.homeopathic.com

This site, belonging to Homeopathic Educational Services, is a cornucopia of homeopathic principles, history, research, and self-care. It also includes an extensive catalog of quality books, CD-ROMs, instructional tapes, and even correspondence courses. For a diverting treat, click on "Interesting Stuff."

www.lyghtforce.com

Click on "Homeopathy On-Line Magazine," and there, that is just what you'll find: a cyber magazine devoted to classical home-opathy and modern practice, complete with feature stories, columns, editorials, and book reviews.

www.medicinegarden.com

Click on the "Classical Homeopathy" link and there, among other goodies (like homeopathic quizzes and "Frequently Asked Questions"), you will find the entirety of Hahnemann's *Organon* on-line.

www.nesh.com

This is the site for the New England School of Homeopathy. Here you can find the *New England Journal of Homeopathy,* a semiannual publication which began in 1992 and which focuses each issue on a single topic or remedy. Although it's most relevant to serious students of homeopathy, it is nevertheless worth a visit by the ardent "browser."

www.boiron.fr

Don't panic—though this site first comes up in French, just click on the "English" button for an instantaneous translation. Among other things, you'll find an excellent resource for keeping up with the latest research developments in homeopathy.

www.simillibus.com

Run by a homeopathic M.D., this site contains a plethora of valuable general information and excellent links to the worlds of homeopathic and conventional medicine. There is a great section called "Remedy of the Week," which examines one remedy—sometimes a lesser known one—in detail. For those with a serious, studious bent, a subscription will get you interactive case analysis.

www.simillimum.com

This site rightly describes itself as a cyberspace academy. It offers on-line homeopathic education for the most serious students of classical Hahnemannian homeopathy. Even so, some delights await the dabbler. For example, check out "The Little On-Line Library."

Informative Websites—General Medicine

www.ama-assn.org

This is the Website of the American Medical Association, from which you can access *JAMA* and its numerous other publications. Here, you can keep up with the latest developments in allopathic medicine. The site has a wonderful archive feature to look up past articles of interest. And if you like, you can get on an e-mail list to automatically receive a weekly copy of *JAMA*'s contents.

www.nejm.org

This is the Website of the *New England Journal of Medicine,* another of the most well-respected journals of conventional medicine. This is another avenue for keeping up with new research. However, unlike with *JAMA,* you have to subscribe to get full text articles.

www.queendom.com/medline.html

This Healthgate site offers a link to many excellent medical databases, including Medline, in which you can look up abstracts (and order corresponding full text articles if you wish) on virtually any medical subject that has been covered in a major journal since 1966.

There are also other ways to tap into the Medline database if you wish. Just type "Medline" into your favorite Internet search engine.

www.rxlist.com

Visit this site to investigate the effects—and side effects—of any prescription drug. Simply do a keyword search, either by generic or brand name.

Repertories and Materia Medica

There are many repertories to choose from, but most of the "classics"—such as J. T. Kent's repertory, which is widely used by professionals—are written in language we would consider somewhat antiquated and, hence, confusing.

For a full-fledged repertory written in modern language and arranged in a user-friendly fashion try:

Homeopathic Medical Repertory
By Robin Murphy, N.D.
(Second Edition, 1996)
Publisher: The Hahnemann Academy of North America,
Durango, CO

As a beginner, you may also want one book that conveniently includes both a brief repertory and a materia medica, both relating to the most common ailments and remedies you are likely to encounter. For this I recommend a very affordable paperback:

The People's Repertory
By Luc De Schepper, M.D., Ph.D., C.Hom.
Publisher: Full of Life Publishing, Santa Fe, NM, 1998

If you are going to delve a bit deeper into homeopathy, you may want to look at, and perhaps own, an in-depth materia medica. My favorite, both for format and content, is:

The Essentials of Homeopathic Materia Medica
By Jacques Jouanny, M.D.
Publisher: Editions Boiron, France, 1995

For one last addition to your bag of tricks, try the pocket-sized combination repertory/materia medica that, in earlier editions, was carried by homeopaths on house calls for nearly a century. It's convenient yet thorough, and—-as my neighbor successfully hinted to her husband last year—makes a great Mother's Day gift.

Materia Medica with Repertory
By William Boericke, M.D.
(Ninth Edition, 1927)
Publisher: Boericke & Tafel, Inc., Santa Rosa, CA

Other Useful and Informative Books

For good introductory overviews, take a look at the following:

Patient's Guide to Homeopathic Medicine
By Judyth Reichenberg-Ullman, N.D., and Robert Ullman, N.D.
Picnic Point Press: 1994

The Consumer's Guide to Homeopathy
By Dana Ullman, M.P.H.
Tarcher/Putnam: 1995

Homeopathy: Beyond Flat Earth Medicine
By Timothy Dooley, N.D., M.D.
Timing Publications: 1995

Demystifying Homeopathy
By Jacob Mirman, M.D.
New Hope Publishers: 1997

Human Condition Critical
By Dr. Luc De Schepper, M.D., Ph.D., C.Hom.
Full of Life Publishing: 1993

Here are some excellent books on self-care and home care—though they are not meant to replace appropriate professional medical consultation.

Healing with Homeopathy: The Doctor's Guide
By Wayne Jonas M.D., and Jennifer Jacobs, M.D.
Warner: 1998

The Complete Homeopathy Handbook
By Miranda Castro
St. Martin's: 1991

Homeopathic Medicine at Home
By Maesimund Panos, M.D., and Jane Heimlich
Tarcher: 1981

These books specialize in childbirth and infant care:

Homeopathic Medicines for Pregnancy and Childbirth
By Richard Moskowitz, M.D.
North Atlantic Books: 1992

Homeopathy for Pregnancy, Birth and the First Year
By Miranda Castro
St. Martin's: 1993

These books specialize in constitutional types:

The Homeopathic Treatment of Children: Pediatric Constitutional Types
By Paul Herscu, M.D.
North Atlantic Books: 1991

*Homeopathic Psychology: Personality Profiles of the Major
Constitutional Remedies*
By Philip Bailey, M.D.
North Atlantic Books: 1996

Here is a book for those of you who don't want to leave anyone
in the family out:

Homeopathic Care for Cats and Dogs
By Donald Hamilton, D.V.M.
North Atlantic Books: 1999

Here are some books for more advanced study. They delve into
science, philosophy, and practice in greater depth than the above.
Still, they are accessible to the interested general reader.

Homeopathy: The Great Riddle
By Richard Grossinger
North Atlantic Books: 1980

The Science of Homeopathy
By George Vithoulkas and William A. Tiller
Grove Press: 1980

Here are some excellent books on the use of homeopathy for developmental and emotional issues:

Ritalin-Free Kids
By Judyth Reichenberg-Ullman, N.D., and Robert Ullman, N.D.
Prima Publishing: 1996

Prozac-Free
By Judyth Reichenberg-Ullman, N.D., and Robert Ullman, N.D.
Prima Publishing: 1999

Here are two books on the practices, and some of the pitfalls, of conventional medicine which are easy to read, and very eye-opening:

Breaking the Antibiotic Habit
By Paul A. Offit, M.D., Bonne Fass-Offit, M.D., and Louis Bell, M.D.
John Wiley & Sons: 1999

How to Raise a Healthy Child in Spite of Your Doctor
By Robert S. Mendelsohn, M.D.
Ballantine: 1984

Lastly, here are two fine books on alternative approaches which include, but are not exclusive to, homeopathy.

Radical Healing
By Rudolph Ballantine, M.D.
Harmony Books: 1999

Spontaneous Healing
By Andrew Weil, M.D.
Knopf: 1995

Where to Find Books

In addition to general-interest bookstores, health food stores and pharmacies are carrying more and more books on homeopathy. However, if you have any difficulty locating the books listed in the foregoing sections, or if you want to inquire about any other books, here are two mail-order services that have comprehensive inventories and knowledgeable staffs:

Minimum Price Books
Blaine, Washington
1-800-663-8272 (orders)
604-597-4757 (inquiries)
E-mail: orders@minimum.com
Website: www.minimum.com

Homeopathic Educational Services
Berkeley, CA
1-800-359-9051 (orders)
510-649-0294 (inquiries, catalog requests*)
E-mail: mail@homeopathic.com
Website: www.homeopathic.com

*Order a catalog; it is great fun to browse.

Software

Computers and homeopathy are a wonderful match, and not surprisingly, most of the information in repertories and materia medica has been cross-referenced, and put onto CD-ROMs. For professionals, extensive programs that cost in excess of $1000 are available, and are more and more commonly used. Obviously, it's unlikely you will want to make this much of an investment—and it's not necessary for basic home care.

There are, however, some CD-ROMs that are comparatively inexpensive (under $100) which are useful—and fun if you enjoy working on your computer. They allow you, for example, to make lists of symptoms and have the program do the work of finding corresponding remedies. Check out:

The Jacobs Homeopathic Prescriber
Developed by Jennifer Jacobs, M.D., M.P.H.

Many beginners find this easy to use because it is based on Western classifications of illness but then tailored to each person's unique symptom picture.

The Homeopathic Resource
(Also available on disk)

This is a more repertory-based program; you look up individual symptoms the way you would in a repertory book. There's a bit more of a "learning curve" when it comes to using it, but users love it.

If you become a bit more advanced, and are willing to invest a bit more money, try one of these two programs (between $150 and $200):

The Ozone Program

The Homeopathic Educational Services catalog describes this as "the next step up" for those who want to prescribe quickly and accurately in an individualized fashion. It includes all of Kent's and Boericke's repertories, which is pretty impressive for the price.

The Gift of Homeopathy
Developed by MacRepertory

This is the program I use, and I really enjoy it. In addition to Kent's repertory and a materia medica, it includes several books of homeopathic philosophy. It also has great graphics and—best of all—works on my Mac. A nice feature: When you buy it, $100 goes to homeopathic organizations.

Two caveats when it comes to purchasing and using these programs. First, make sure that whatever you purchase is compatible with your computer and operating system. Second, don't imagine any computer program can point you to the right remedy if you don't do a good, thorough job of observing and inputing symptoms. As they say in computer lingo: garbage in, garbage out.

Suppliers

It is getting increasingly easy to find a wide selection of homeopathic remedies in pharmacies as well as in health food stores. You may never have the need to order remedies on your own, but if you do, here are two sources I rely on and trust:

HOMEOPATHY OVERNIGHT
1-800-ARNICA30
www.homeopathyovernight.com

NATURAL HEALTH SUPPLY
1-888-689-1608 or
505-474-9175
www.A2Zhomeopathy.com

A MEDICINE MOM'S GLOSSARY OF HOMEOPATHY

acute, self-limiting condition A medical situation that has intense, disturbing symptoms (e.g., flus, colds, diarrhea) but is generally of short duration and will, in most cases, ultimately correct itself.

aggravation A situation in which symptoms worsen after taking a remedy. Over all, this can be a positive indication, as it means the remedy is probably the right one. But even though the aggravation will likely pass and lead to healing, it can be unsettling for someone with little or no experience in homeopathy. Probably the potency is too high or the remedy is being given too frequently, and adjustments should be made.

allopathy Throughout this book this phrase has been used to denote conventional Western medicine—its approach and philosophy. Allopathy tends to treat symptoms with agents that induce opposite effects, e.g., treating congestion with a decongestant. Allopathy is not a bad word, but is a very different approach from homeopathy, which treats like with like.

alternative medicine A catch-all phrase which is often used to encompass any medical interventions that are not part of the prevailing, orthodox system of health care. With more and more aspects of so-called alternative systems becoming mainstreamed, the term is likely to give way to "complementary" or "integrative" medicine.

Avogadro's number A mathematical constant; the water dilution level of 12C (or its equivalent, 24X), above which no molecule of the original substance remains present in physical form.

Bach flower remedies Flower essences said to work on moods, temperaments, and emotions. Many people think these are homeopathic, but strictly speaking they are not—however, some homeopathic practitioners integrate them in treatment.

chronic condition A health condition that is long-lasting and not self-resolving, e.g., psoriasis, arthritis. Homeopathy can be especially effective in dealing with chronic conditions, but never try to treat a chronic condition yourself, homeopathically or otherwise.

classical homeopath In general, a homeopath who only administers one remedy at a time, carefully selecting it to fit the overall symptom picture.

combination remedy A homeopathic remedy that blends a group of remedies proven, on an individual basis, to be effective for a common condition (e.g., hayfever, sinusitus). The upside to these combinations is that they may work well enough for some people and some conditions and do not require that one try to find an appropriate individual remedy. The downside is that an individualized remedy can work even more quickly and effectively, and on a deeper level. On balance, combinations may be helpful for beginners who might otherwise feel confused.

complementary medicine This generally refers to the integration of so-called alternative therapies with traditional allopathy.

constitution The entirety of a person's emotional, mental, and physical makeup, including their temperament, behavior, appearance, strengths, and frailties.

constitutional remedy The homeopathic remedy corresponding to a person's constitutional type, and of fundamental importance to the overall well-being of the individual. Usually, the constitutional remedy is not given until any acute conditions have cleared.

dilution The number of times a minute amount of a remedy's original substance has been dissolved in water.

generalities In homeopathic lingo, these are symptom traits that apply to the overall person, i.e., "I feel better in the cool night air," or "I am always depressed in the autumn." Generalities, especially ones that have to do with a person's emotional state, can offer critical information in case-taking, and a homeopath will usually ask many questions concerning them during intake.

genus epidemicus This is the term for a group of the most prevalent symptoms of a large number of people afflicted with a contagious disease, e.g., a flu epidemic. Once this is known, the "remedy epidemicus" can be found.

Hahnemann, Samuel The founder of homeopathy, a German born physician and pharmacist (1755–1843).

Hering's Law (of Cure) The idea that, during homeopathic treatment symptoms disappear in an orderly fashion, with the most recently acquired ones being reversed before the longer-embedded ones.

integrative medicine See complementary medicine, although this term is newer and really seems to be catching on with doctors.

isopathy A remedy that is not a "similar" but a "same," for example one might take *apis*—which is made from the honeybee—to treat a bee sting. Although the remedy is prepared homeopathically, it is technically an isopathic remedy.

Law of Similars *Similia similibus curantur,* which is Latin for "Like shall be cured by like," is the most fundamental doctrine of homeopathy, which employs remedies that would, in a well person, induce symptoms similar to those being experienced by an unwell person (e.g., a remedy made from red onion is used to treat watery nose and eyes).

Law of the Minimum Dose The other fundamental tenet of homeopathy, it originated when Hahnemann discovered that infinitesimal doses of similars had beneficial actions, with diminishing side effects.

LM potency A potency experimented with and written about by Hahnemann late in his career. The LM potency—which requires complex preparation and should be taken under a practitioner's guidance—is actually a gentle, low dose, but works with the efficacy of a high dose.

Materia medica Literally "medical matter," and the branch of science which studies drugs and doses. In homeopathy, it is a reference work listing remedies and their corresponding therapeutic actions.

mother tincture The initial liquid from which homeopathic remedies are made.

naturopathy (or naturopathic medicine) A system of medicine that generally integrates such elements as herbology, homeopathy, acupuncture, soft tissue manipulations, nutritional guidance, and supplements. Naturopathic physicians are called N.D.s, and are currently licensed in at least a dozen states (see the Resource Section).

NWS (never well since) Sometimes a person's health will take a turn for the worse following a particular physical or emotional event (e.g., following an operation or vaccination; or following a divorce or death in the family). During case-taking, a homeopath will attempt to determine if there is a NWS factor, and tailor remedies accordingly.

Organon Hahnemann's *magnum opus,* which included extensive information on conducting homeopathic treatment and preparing remedies. *The Organon* went through six editions.

osteopath Physicians whose names are followed by D.O., instead of M.D., are osteopathic physicians. Although this appellation originally indicated they had all the standard medical training plus additional training in manipulations of the spine and joints, many contemporary osteopaths practice no differently than M.D.s. As far as insurers are concerned, an M.D. and a D.O. are virtually the same entity, and both degrees carry equal prestige. If you want an osteopath who actually integrates aspects of osteopathy in practice, initials alone won't tell you what you need to know, so ask.

otitis media Middle ear infection, sometimes referred to as acute otitis media (AOM).

placebo A substance given to patients which itself is inert (e.g., a sugar pill), but which the patient may believe has curative powers.

plussing A method of extending the amount—and slightly increasing the potency—of a liquid homeopathic remedy by adding more water. There are many variations of this method, so do as your practitioner advises.

polychrest A remedy with many widespread uses, works on mental, emotional and physical levels, and is used to treat chronic as well as acute disorders. Some examples of polychrests are *Arsenicum album, Natrum muriaticum,* and *Nux vomica.*

potency The strength of a homeopathic remedy, generally represented by a number and letter (e.g., 6C, 12X, or 30C) which indicate to what degree a remedy has been diluted and succussed.

proving The process by which homeopathic remedies are tested on healthy subjects by noting and recording what symptoms are induced. When the same substances are given to an ill person displaying such symptoms, the symptoms should reverse, according to the Law of Similars.

remedy Homeopathic medicines are called "remedies" as opposed to drugs. According to Hahnemann, a "drug" merely induces an illness—i.e., an unbalanced state—of its own, which temporarily overshadows the original symptoms but does not truly foster healing. A remedy, on the other hand, actually remedies a situation by allowing the body to heal itself.

repertory In homeopathy, an index of symptoms.

rubric A class or category, as in a category of symptoms. A repertory is a collection of rubrics.

simillimum This word translates as "the most similar." In homeopathy, it refers to the "bull's-eye" remedy, which matches the symptom picture so precisely it results in rapid and complete healing.

small remedy This refers to a remedy that works very specifically on just a few symptoms. It may be used frequently (e.g., *calendula* for sunburn and skin irritation), but not for the broad range of ailments a polychrest would work on.

succussion The process of shaking with impact (e.g., thumping against a hard surface) a diluted homeopathic remedy, in order to strengthen it.

symptom According to homeopathic theory, an expression of the body's attempt to correct an underlying imbalance.

symptom picture An individual's totality of symptoms: physical, mental, and emotional.

tissue salts (also known as cell salts) Twelve low-potency remedies developed by German homeopathic physician W. H. Schuessler, which have been incorporated into the homeopathic materia medica. They are prepared from minerals already present in the body and have specific, gentle, healing effects on the body's tissues.

water method The process of diluting a homeopathic tablet or pellet in water, so that it may be administered in liquid form. An effective way of giving remedies to small children, and of making your remedies longer-lasting and more portable (by carrying them around in small plastic water bottles). Follow your practitioner's suggestions as to amounts of remedy and added water.

A QUICK GUIDE TO HOMEOPATHIC POTENCIES

Most of the potencies you see on homeopathic remedies will probably consist of a number (e.g., 6, 12, 30, 200) followed by a C. On occasion, however, the number may be followed by an X. The X means the remedy was prepared using a different scale of water to original substance. Without getting into a convoluted mathematical explanation, all you need to know as a consumer is that a "C" potency is equivalent to its double in an X potency. So, for example:

$$3C = 6X$$
$$6C = 12X$$
$$12C = 24X$$

and so on.

Here is how the potencies are generally used:

3C (or 6X)   This is usually the potency of a tissue salt. Tissue salts (aka, cell salts) are very gentle low-potency remedies prepared from common minerals found in the human body. They work well on the cells and tissues of the body, and are used for treating such conditions as inflammations and edema, among other things.

6C   This is a common, safe potency that you will find in a
             drugstore or health food store. It is generally used to
             treat chronic conditions—though your practitioner
             may give you special instructions for use in some
             acute cases. In 6C there is still a small (very, very
             small) trace of the original substance in the remedy.

12C   Sometimes you will find this in stores, though not as
             readily as you will 6C or 30C. Some consider it a
             middle ground, a good pick if you are not sure
             whether to use a 6C or a 30C. Above this point—
             which is Avogadro's number—no molecule of the
             original substance remains present in molecular form
             in the remedy.

30C   This is the most commonly used potency, and the eas-
             iest to find. 30C is used to treat acute, self-limiting
             conditions, e.g., colds, ear infections, allergic reac-
             tions, and stomach upset.

200C   If you are a beginner, do not administer potencies
             above 30C. A 200C potency can be extremely effec-
             tive, but may also have the potential to aggravate, es-
             pecially if given too often. Once you know what you
             are doing, have had some instruction, and consulted a
             professional, you may wish to use this potency on oc-
             casion. (Sometimes, one dose of it may even be used
             as a preventative.) Generally this potency is not on
             display, but often a pharmacy will have it stocked be-
             hind the counter.

1M   Now we are really getting into high potencies. On oc-
             casion a professional homeopath may advise you to
             use a 1M. Some individuals actually find it more ef-

fective than 200C, but some are too sensitive to take it.

10M   This potency is used almost exclusively for constitutionals. Always consult a professional for administering constitutionals.

LM   This potency was used by Hahnemann late in his career, and many classical homeopaths consider it his crowning achievement. LMs are actually low-potency remedies; however, I list them on this end of the scale because they work as effectively as high-potency ones while rarely causing aggravations—since they are so gentle. A constitutional may also be administered in an LM dosage, in liquid form.

SOME COMMON KIDS' CONSTITUTIONAL TYPES

The following pages offer "thumbnail sketches" of some of the most common children's constitutional types. This is for the purposes of information, understanding, and fun (I always find it enjoyable to speculate on such categorizations regarding family members and friends). However, I think it's important to restate here that constitutional remedies should be administered only under the guidance of a homeopath. In addition, do not be surprised if a homeopath comes up with a different "type" than you did. There are many nuances to consider, and indeed there are even some less common types of constitutional categories which are not covered here. Besides, as you know, homeopaths pride themselves on studying each case individually and thoroughly. That is the strength—indeed the very basis—of the homeopathic method.

The Sulphur Type

If you have a baby or a toddler who is already showing signs of intense curiosity and burgeoning independence, you may well have a Sulphur child. Another clue to their "Sulphurhood" is that they hate to have their diapers changed. They don't mind being dirty, especially if it means they can go on doing whatever it was they were doing before you started to pester them.

Still another tipoff is that Sulphurs are "warm-blooded." They always seem to kick their covers off at night (or at least stick their feet out from underneath the blankets). When you pick them up from a sound sleep, they are warm as toast. Last but not least, you might recognize Sulphurs by the fact that they have a great deal of excess energy just before bedtime (whee!).

As Sulphurs get a bit older, you will often find them being "leader of the pack." Although they might not be the best at sports, they are always the one organizing the game (and adding some special "rules" of their own). Friends to everyone, they will always encourage all the kids to join in—even the shy loners who might otherwise stay on the sidelines.

Sulphurs are quite intelligent. They incorporate new information quickly, and their motor skills are good. They have a way with words and can talk just about anyone into anything, without the other party knowing what hit them. (Future lawyers and politicians, no doubt.) However, they are often loath to take advice or instruction from others, and can get frustrated and irritable if there is something they cannot quickly master on their own.

That infantile tendency to stay in dirty diapers never exactly goes away for Sulphurs. It transforms into a general messiness and disarray. In fact, let's put it this way: Personal hygiene, overall, is not their strong suit.

Sulphurs can also be somewhat self-centered. But they are so dynamic and personable, they often get away with this (a bit too much, some might say!). They can have volatile tempers, but cool down quickly and never hold grudges. And they are notoriously quick wits.

As teens, Sulphurs are often prone to acne. And throughout their lives—because of their *bon vivant* tendencies and cravings for rich and spicy foods—they may require various digestive remedies. They need to monitor all their sensual cravings carefully too, because they can be prone to addictions. Another physical problem they may be prone to—from childhood onward—is respiratory ailments.

As an adult, your Sulphur child will likely be ambitious and competitive (maybe a workaholic if they don't make a conscious effort to relax now and again).

In general, where Sulphurs are concerned, there is rarely a dull moment—for them or for their parents.

The Pulsitilla Type

As opposed to the independent-minded Sulphur baby, the Pulsitilla infant is a clinger and a "burrower" where their parents are concerned. They can simply never get too close, and can lose their cool if their mom so much as walks across the room or, heaven forbid, into the next one. They often will not go to sleep unless nursed and rocked (or unless a parent lies down beside them). Needless to say, these children are not big fans of weaning. They'd like to be breastfed, well . . . forever.

The Pulsitilla child is bashful, but very affectionate and endearing. Pulsitillas are always seeking approval, and usually get it because they are eager to please—and have figured out just how to keep those hugs and kisses coming. If you are the parent of a Pulsitilla child, however, be prepared for some potential traumas on first days of school. And if younger siblings are born into the family, be prepared for older Pulsitillas to arrange to be "babied" as well. They may, for example, begin to wet the bed again, or even fall prey to an ailment with psychosomatic roots.

Pulsitillas can be weepy, and have a great deal of difficulty making decisions about anything. At their worst, Pulsitillas can be jealous and possessive. It will be a parent's challenge (and a homeopath's) to help them moderate these tendencies and to give and receive love in a more balanced fashion.

Pulsitillas are prone to ear infections (acute otitis media), to sinusitis, and to croup and bronchitis (and even pneumonia). They often come down with a lot of colds, and have allergies. When Pulsitilla girls start their menses, they are prone to emotional PMS symptoms.

As you may have inferred from all this, parents of a Pulsitilla child might do very well bringing that child to a homeopath early in their development to mitigate some of these tendencies.

The Calcarea Carbonica (Calc Carb) Type

Many children in this country are born as this type, though some may evolve into a different constitutional type later on. Calc carb babies are the "oochie coochie coo" kind. They are happy little chubba-bubbas with substantially pinchable cheeks. It's pretty easy to tell if you have one of these cutie pies, especially because they tend to alternate between days of constipation and astonishingly prolific bowel movements that will set you back a fortune in wet wipes. They also tend to spit up a lot (more wet wipes!) and to hiccough. Diaper rash is also common.

As Calc carbs grow, they are classic late bloomers. Their fontanels are late to close, and they are often the last to teethe, walk, and talk. (Don't worry—they will get there!) They also tend to be chilly, and they tire out easily.

Although they do not tend to volunteer the answers when at school (and so may sometimes be overlooked or underrated by teachers), Calc carbs tend to be quite bright, with impressive powers of logic and concentration.

Calc carb children tend to be cautious, and they can elevate worrying to an art form. They are also easily affected by anything they may see on television, so be forewarned: you will want to monitor their television fare closely. In addition, they don't like the dark, and are prone to night terrors.

Calc carbs are good-natured and good at sharing. Their fine

sense of humor makes them love to tease (but they are not so good at being teased). Though inwardly sensitive, they can behave with stubbornness and obstinacy on the outside. They are also great homebodies. Don't expect them to be overjoyed at the prospect of, say, summer camp. And be prepared for their emotional turmoil if you move to a new house.

In addition to being constipation-prone, Calc carbs are prone to ear infections, eczema, canker sores, and headaches (from mental strain and eye strain). They may have runny noses even when healthy.

Calc carbs are carbohydrate cravers, and have less than efficient metabolisms. Hence the chubbiness that marked their childhood may be a lifelong problem for them if they remain this constitutional type. Although many do remain this type for their entire lives, some evolve into other types at puberty and may end up tall and lean.

Here's an interesting note: For those who do remain Calc carbs, their nature (sympathetic, home-loving, generous to friends and family) tends to make them wonderful parents in adulthood.

The Phosphorus Type

Phosphorus types are beautiful babies, with bright eyes and long lashes, and fine skin and features. They are usually a bit thin for their length but still quite adorable and huggable, as they are happy and good-natured from the get-go. Phosphorus infants hate loud, sudden noises, and they love their refreshing naps (as they probably will throughout life).

The growing Phosphorus child is extroverted and expressive. Though Phosphorus types are excitable, on the whole they have very good manners.

Phosphorus kids have a good rapport with just about everyone, and like Sulphurs, you will often find them leading the neighborhood games (though in their case it is because their enthusiasm is so infectious). They hate to be thought of as average, and believe they can master any task even if it is beyond their years.

The Phosphorus type is very curious, and often has an artistic bent and a talent for painting, singing, drama, or dance. Basically, Phosphorus is beautiful and loves beautiful things. This type also enjoys dressing well, and shows a flair for fashion.

Phosphorus types love to be the center of attention, and sometimes their communication skills tend to go a bit overboard. They may talk for a *loooonnng* time, and at a somewhat high volume (look at me!). As adults, Phosphorus types will demand lots and lots of attention from their romantic partners, and if this is not forthcoming, they may find themselves in and out of relationships.

Phosphorus is very empathic, very spiritual, and also very sensitive. A Phosphorus will pick up on, and absorb (sometimes to their detriment) whatever is in their immediate surroundings—from good or bad "vibes" to airborne chemicals, toxins and pollens. As you can imagine, this predisposes them to hay fever and various bronchial ailments, as well as to headaches that develop from smelling strong odors. They tend not to have a lot of stamina (so remember their need for those refreshing naps). And they also are prone to many fears, such as fear of the dark, fear of insects, and the vague fear that something bad may happen.

All in all, I think of Phosphorus as a flower—heartwarming, lovely, inspiring, fragile.

The Natrum Muriaticum (Nat mur) Type

Not that many infants begin life in a Nat mur state—which is basically a sad or depressed state. Those who do generally have mothers who experience sadness or loss during their pregnancy, or are separated from their mothers at birth (perhaps because they are premature and need to spend time in an incubator). Babies who are

Nat mur tend to be pale, even anemic looking. They cry little and do not much care to be handled. As toddlers they are late to walk and talk, but usually early to toilet-train because they like cleanliness.

For the most part, children develop a Nat mur constitution a bit later on in childhood, often between the ages of four and six. This may be due to an overt trauma that causes grief (e.g., a death in the family or a divorce) or to subtler, but very powerful forces (e.g., being bullied and picked on by other children).

Nat mur types are not resilient, but rather hang on to their hurts. With each rejection, they will become more dejected, and isolate themselves more. Since this worsens their sense of loneliness, this is an unfortunate cycle. It *is* a cycle that can often be broken, with the help of concerned parents, professional assistance, and the constitutional remedy that can counteract the Nat mur characteristics of withdrawal and retention (i.e., retention of grievances, and the holding back of unspilt tears).

However, if the cycle keeps going on, the person who will likely develop is an adolescent and, later, an adult haunted by heartbreaks and betrayals—as well as by feeling guilt because they think "it is all their fault." Sometimes, however, in adulthood, the great empathy that Nat mur types develop for other sufferers lead them to excel in fields such as counseling and psychotherapy, or to become tireless crusaders for the underdog. Still, in these endeavors they must be careful not to martyr themselves.

On the physical side, the Nat mur type is prone to insomnia, headaches, dry mouth, and frequent canker sores. Many are myopic from a young age. They suffer when being exposed to direct sunlight. They crave salts and sweets, and are often somewhat overweight, both from diet and metabolism—as well as from retaining water. But I have known Nat mur types who successfully lost weight and kept it off for the first time after being given their constitutional.

The Silicea Type

Silicea babies and children are primarily Nordic types, with light skin and hair, and blue eyes. For all its loveliness, though, their fine hair falls out easily, and their nails are brittle as well. Their posture is a little stooped and they are late walkers. They are picky eaters but always thirsty, and they frequently feel chilly. Many of them have trouble digesting milk.

These children are very capable, and also very organized, but they tend to lack self-confidence and are afraid they will fail. They easily cry when scolded, and they don't like to be comforted afterward, preferring to nurse their grievances alone. Although generally timid, at times they can become quite cross.

The delicate skin of a Silicea is prone to infections, as well as to warts, pimples, and other eruptions. Their eyes are also subject to inflammations, and Siliceas tend to suffer from headaches attended by nausea.

As adults, Siliceas still tend to suffer confidence problems, even if they are not warranted based on their skills. For example, they are terrified of speaking in public, but do just fine when they force themselves to face their fears.

The Lycopodium Type

Lycopodium infants are fearful and anxious. They hate being around strangers (i.e., anyone other than a parent). They are cranky and cry a lot (especially when hungry, and between 4 P.M. and 8 P.M.). From the start, the parents immediately sense the great demands this child is placing upon them.

The heads of these babies may seem a bit large in proportion to their bodies. From birth they may have eczema and many colds. Indeed, they always seem to be sniffling.

Some Lycopodiums may have difficulty developing the sucking reflex, but once they start sucking their thumb, they may do this for many years.

Lycopodium types will continue being anxious and apprehensive as they grow. They do not like trying new things. Often parents will comment that Lycopodium children have flat affects, and never seem very enthusiastic about anything.

One thing Lycopodiums do like, though, is personal power. They are bossy and impatient, and tend to order even their parents around. Toward siblings, the Lycopodium child can be quite manipulative. They generally prefer playing only with younger kids, so they can call all the shots.

Lycopodiums may have difficulty sorting out left from right, and are prone to dyslexia. Mistakes they make in reading and arithmetic frustrate them greatly. Most Lycopodiums are restless, and some are hyperactive.

Lycopodiums can't stand to be criticized (they get moody and weepy), but do tend to find fault with others. If left unchecked and untreated, this tendency expands as they reach adolescence.

Lycopodiums crave sweets, and are frequently constipated. They are prone to headaches that result from hunger, to sore throats and tonsilitis, to dry cracked skin, and to mononucleosis. Many of their physical aches and pains tend to start on the right side, and then move to the left.

REFERENCES

Introduction

1. Eisenberg, DM, Davis, RB, Ettner, SL, et al. Trends in alternative medicine use in the United States, 1990–97. *Journal of the American Medical Association,* 1998; 280:1569–75.
2. Jacobs, J, Chapman, EH, Crothers, D. Patient characteristics and practice patterns of physicians using homeopathy. *Archives of Archives of Family Medicine,* 1998; 7:537–40.

Chapter 1

1. In a letter to William James, September 27, 1890, published in *The Diary of Alice James,* ed. Leon Edel (1964).
2. Ballantine, Rudolph. *Radical Healing* (New York: Harmony Books, 1999), p. 72.
3. "So Listen to Your Mother Already; For Flu Take Chicken Soup." *The New York Times,* February 3, 1999, p. F5.
4. Mendelsohn, Robert S. *How to Raise a Healthy Child . . . in Spite of Your Doctor* (New York: Ballantine, 1984).

Chapter 2

1. Thomas, Lewis. *The Lives of a Cell: Notes of a Biology Watcher* (New York: Viking, 1974), p. 72. (Italics added by this author.)
2. Cited in Steven Locke and Douglas Colligan. *The Healer Within* (New York: Dutton, 1986), p. 25.
3. Thomas, op. cit., pp. 88–89.
4. For a fascinating read on this topic, see Larry Dossey, M.D. *Healing Words: The Power of Prayer and the Practice of Medicine* (San Francisco: HarperCollins, 1993).
5. Pichichero, M.E. Changing the treatment paradigm for acute otitis media in children. *Journal of the American Medical Association,* 1998; 279:1748–50.
6. Kozyrskyj, AL, Hildes-Ripstein, GE, Longstaffe, JL, et. al. Treatment of acute otitis media with a shortened course of antibiotics: a meta-analysis. *Journal of the American Medical Association,* 1998; 279:1736–42.
7. Pichichero, op. cit.
8. For a detailed overview of antibiotic side effects, see Dr. Mary Ann Block's book *No More Amoxicillin* (New York: Kensington, 1998).
9. Ibid., p. 149.
10. "Losing the Battle of the Bugs." *U.S. News & World Report,* p. 52–58 (May 10, 1999).
11. Ibid., p. 58.
12. Offit, PA, Fass-Offit, B., Bell, L. *Breaking the Antibiotic Habit.* (New York: Wiley, 1999), pp. 62–63.
13. *U.S. News & World Report,* op. cit., p. 58.
14. Konner, Melvin. *Becoming a Doctor: A Journey of Initiation in Medical School* (New York: Viking, 1987), p. 366.
15. The study, originally reported in *Pediatrics,* was cited in *U.S. News & World Report,* op. cit.

Chapter 3

1. Stephanopoulos, George. *All Too Human* (New York: Little, Brown, 1999), p. 297.
2. A detailed history of homeopathy in the United States is chronicled in Harris Coulter's book, *Divided Legacy: The Conflict Between Homeopathy and the American Medical Association* (Berkeley: North

Atlantic, 1981). This is actually the third of four volumes in Coulter's magnum opus, *Divided Legacy: A History of the Schism in Modern Medical Thought.*

3. This study, by P. C. Endler, W. Pongrantz, and G. Kastberg, et al, was published in *Veterinary and Human Toxicology,* 1994, 36:56.
4. Friese, KH, Kruse, S, Moeller, H. Acute otitis media in children: a comparison of homeopathic and conventional treatment. *Biomedical Therapy,* 1997; 60, 4:113–16 (originally published in German in *Head, Nose, Throat Otolyngarology,* August 1996: 462–66).
5. Jacobs, J, Jimenez, LM, Gloyd, SS, et al. Treatment of acute childhood diarrhea with homeopathic medicine: a randomized clinical trial in Nicaragua. *Pediatrics,* May 1994; 93, 5:719–25.
6. Reilly, D, Taylor, M, McSherry, C. Is homeopathy a placebo response? Controlled trial of homeopathic potency with pollen in hayfever as model. *Lancet,* October 18, 1986; 881–86.
7. Reilly, D, Taylor, M, Beattie, N, et al. Is evidence for homeopathy reproducible? *Lancet,* December 10, 1994; 344:1601–6.
8. Linde, K, Clausius, N, Ramirez, G, et al. Are the clinical effects of homeopathy placebo effects? A meta-analysis of placebo controlled trials. *Lancet,* September 20, 1997; 350:834–43.
9. Kleijnen, J, Knipschild, P, ter Riet, G. Clinical trials of homeopathy. *British Medical Journal,* February 9, 1991; 302:316–23.
10. Marvel, MK, Epstein, RM, Flowers, K, et. al. Soliciting the patient's agenda: have we improved? *Journal of the American Medical Association,* 1999; 281:283–87.
11. Jacons, J, Chapman, E, Crothers, D. Patient Characteristics and Practice Patterns of Physicians Using Homeopathy. *Archives of Family Medicine,* 1998; 7:537–40.

Chapter 4

1. "Homeopathy in the USA." American Homeopathic Pharmaceutical Association. 1995–96, pp. 1–8.
2. Eisenberg, DM, Davis, RB, Ettner, SL, et al. Trends in alternative medicine use in the United States, 1990–97. *Journal of the American Medical Association,* 1998; 280:1569–75.
3. Jacobs, J. Homeopathic research: Two steps forward, one step back. *Homeopathy Today.* July/August 1999, pp. 13–15.

4. Offit, PA, Fass-Offit, B., Bell, L. *Breaking the Antibiotic Habit* (New York: J. Wiley, 1999), p. 9.
5. "Death by Prescription." *The New York Times,* June 3, 1999, p. 1.

Chapter 7

1. "Americans Mingle Complementary Techniques with Traditional Medical Services, Survey Shows." *Business Wire,* September 18, 1998.
2. Eisenberg, DM, Davis, RB, Ettner, SL, et al. Trends in alternative medicine use in the United States, 1990–97. *Journal of the American Medical Association,* 1998; 280:1569–75.
3. Studdert, DM, Eisenberg, DM, Miller, FH, et al. Medical malpractice implications of alternative medicine. *Journal of the American Medical Association,* 1998; 280:1610–15.
4. Block, Mary Ann. *No More Amoxicillin* (New York: Kensington, 1998), p. 17.

Chapter 8

1. Eisenberg, DM, Davis, RB, Ettner, SL, et al. Trends in alternative medicine use in the United States, 1990–97. *Journal of the American Medical Association,* 1998; 280:1569–75.
2 Eisenberg et al., op. cit.
3. According to the Health Care Financing Administration.
4. Jacobs, J, Chapman, EH, Crothers, D. Patient characteristics and practice patterns of physicians using homeopathy. *Archives of Archives of Family Medicine,* 1998; 7:537–40.
5. "The Benefits of Natural Health Care." *Minneapolis Star Tribune,* October 10, 1998.
6. *Caisse Nationale de l'Assurance Maladie des Travailleurs Salaris,* 1996. As reported on the National Center for Homeopathy Website (www.homeopathic.org/cost.htm).
7. "Many Health Benefits Plans Now Include Alternative Care." *Rocky Mountain News,* October 25, 1998.
8. *Introduction to Homeopathic Medicines for Pharmacies.* Boiron Institute.
9. Ibid.

Chapter 9

1. Lamoni, J. Homeopathic treatment of attention deficit hyperactivity disorder, a controlled study. *British Homeopathic Journal,* 1997, 86:196–200.

INDEX